Putting Your Pet First

A Veterinarian's Perspective

John S. Sleasman, DVM, Dipl. ABVP

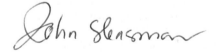

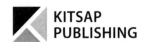

KITSAP
PUBLISHING

Putting Your Pet First: A Veteniarian's Perspective

First edition, published 2016
By John S. Sleasman

Cover Design: RubyRose Neeland
Interior Illustrations: John S. Sleasman
Interior Design & Layout: RubyRose Neeland

ISBN: 978-1-942661-26-9

Published by Kitsap Publishing
19124 Jensen Way NE
P.O. Box 1269
Poulsbo, WA 98370
www.KitsapPublishing.com

Printed in the United States of America

TD 20160331 200-10 9 8 7 6 5 4 3 2 1

CONTENTS

By the end of my childhood years, I believed that the only worth of an animal was in working, producing, or "providing" food on the table. Animals had to have a purpose on the farm. It was simple…or so I thought!

During the 1960s, a special social bond between humans and animals, which likely had existed on some level for eons, was studied and given a name – the human-animal bond. Recognition of this bond and its early days of strengthening began during my veterinary school years. This bond was to change veterinary school curricula and give reason for the escalating advancements and delivery of veterinary pet care that was to follow.

The early years of veterinary practice provide some of my most favorite stories and memories of putting your pet first.

As the client-pet bond strengthens, pet owners turn to pet practitioners for the care of nontraditional pets, as well as cats and dogs.

Big business discovers veterinary medicine. My values from childhood and practice years which built three successful veterinary hospitals now were in direct conflict with the corporate protocols.

The evolution of the human-pet bond is a positive social development. Its evolution has led to medical advancements in veterinary pet care. The rising level of this care has not come without pet owners concerns of affordability, inflexibility, and trust. Lastly, to those concerns I will pose solutions.

PREFACE

Today, for many veterinarians, their professional idealism is being dimmed by the current difficult veterinary business environment. This idealism - often a passionate, childhood calling to help animals - is being overshadowed.

Historically, in the era when a veterinarian 'did it all' in his own private facility, pet owners trusted an unspoken, unwritten professional idealism. Veterinarians were considered and, I say, still are today…humane idealists. Yet, in this modern world, as we see the human-pet bond grow stronger than ever, the effects are directly visible in the veterinary medical field. Yes, it has driven medical skill and knowledge to unbelievable heights in veterinary medicine, which is good. Yet, this tremendous growth in knowledge and skill has exploded into a fragmentation of the veterinary practice delivery system. Specialization is a direct outcome, resulting in the building of separate clinics. Non-profit veterinary facilities are greatly expanding to meet community needs. Emergency clinics are now found in most urban areas. And finally, further adding to the fragmentation, national veterinary corporations with stock holders and investors have entered the veterinary profession in most cities. And yes, we must not forget the 'one doctor' pet practice still alive and the privately owned large group practices. This fragmentation of the veterinary profession contrasts greatly to the passing era when the local veterinarian 'did it all.'

Professional patient and societal obligations, clearly stated within the veterinary oath, are often taking a back seat to business pressures and agendas. For many clients this presents new problems... affordability, inflexible preventative care and treatment protocols, and quite honestly, a question of basic trust.

So let me share a story. The story of why I became a veterinarian with stories of pets as patients, and people as clients in an era when idealism compelled me to become a veterinarian. It includes the troubling changes I personally experienced during my forty years of practice, bringing forth the current realities within the veterinary pet care industry. And finally, I address the current pet owner's angsts with humble solutions in tow. Hopefully, my journey and perspective will serve as a road map to provide you the best care for your pet.

Veterinary Oath

Being admitted to the profession of veterinary medicine, I solemnly swear to use my scientific knowledge and skills for the benefit of society through the protection of animal health and welfare, the prevention and relief of animal suffering, the conservation of animal resources, the promotion of public health, and the advancement of medical knowledge.

I will practice my profession conscientiously, with dignity and in keeping with the principles of veterinary medical ethics.

I accept as a lifelong obligation the continual improvement of my professional knowledge and competence.

Chapter One

Barn Cat Values

"They don't care how much you know till they know how much you care."

- Old Veterinarian's Quote

Lifting the old dog onto the exam table, I remembered her once youthful exuberance. Maggie had been my patient since she was a newborn. Now, as I looked into her soulful eyes, it was time to tell my client that time was passing for his faithful friend. In dog terms, Maggie had certainly lived a charmed life, but even more poignant, she was loved.

Mr. Stanton probably realized the inevitable, but often in a veterinary hospital a client will hope for a medical miracle. I have no magic wand, but professionally, choices can be tailored to the pet and client's needs.

The medical test results indicated the diagnosis had a guarded prognosis. I suggested referring Maggie to a specialist across the Puget Sound, but the client stopped me mid-speech, saying, "No, not only because I really can't afford it, but I don't think that is the best thing for Maggie. You've always been Maggie's vet and I trust you."

Contemplating his concern – appreciating the need for options in a challenging economy – I presented my best treatment plan. Maggie seemed to cock her head. After a minute of quiet reflection, Mr. Stanton asked if he could stay with Maggie for the few days necessary for hospitalization. Surprised at his request, I started my explanation of why that wasn't a practical solution, till a vivid memory interrupted my thoughts. As a boy, waiting the foaling of a mare, I had felt compelled to sleep in the barn. The first step of Maggie's treatment: finding a cot for Mr. Stanton.

It is good to love a pet and be loved by a pet. Mr. Stanton was a fortunate man. Today, I celebrate that relationship, but it wasn't always so. The value of the human-pet bond in our society has evolved through the past decades, and most definitely has become embodied in me. It was my journey: a veterinarian's idealism in a pragmatic world.

In my early years I have no memory of pets, unless one was allowed to count the numerous feral barn cats. The practicality of farm life in the 1940s left little room for sentimentality. A historical time and place were doing their work on my life before I was even born.

My parents were children of the Great Depression. Difficult times were strongly felt by Dad's family in Pacific Beach, a small logging community on the rainy coast of Washington State. Only a decade earlier, the logging industry and tourism boomed in this small coastal town setting. Then the depression hit. Dad was only nineteen years old and lost his job as a logger. The tourism, banks and mills had shut down. There was not a nickel moving in Gray's Harbor County. Families lived on what they scraped together and could harvest from the ocean. Dad was thankful and loyal to President Franklin D. Roosevelt and the Democratic Party, as his administration provided pancake mix, syrup and vitamins to the small ocean community which helped cure boils and other nutritional ailments.

Pets did not seem to be important at this time and place. The only dogs Dad remembered were the beach dogs: strays wandering the beaches and scavenging on dead fish washed up on shore. It must have been a vivid memory because he would often share variations of it with me later in life.

By word of mouth, information circled about a logging job opening in a town twenty-five miles away. There was only one way to make the interview by the next morning. On went the cumbersome logging clothes and down the road he jogged. After traveling throughout the night, his job interview was successful and work began that morning. Dad was the high rigger, a rigorous and dangerous job (Fig. 1).

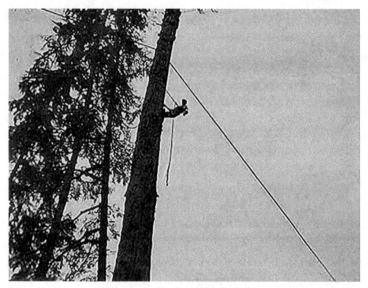

Figure 1: Dad as a high rigger

Loggers didn't have chain saws in those days; they used axes and two-man crosscut timber saws while standing on springboards. When they were falling cedar trees with a thirteen foot diameter, it would take one day to do the undercut and another full day to complete the final cut (Fig. 2).

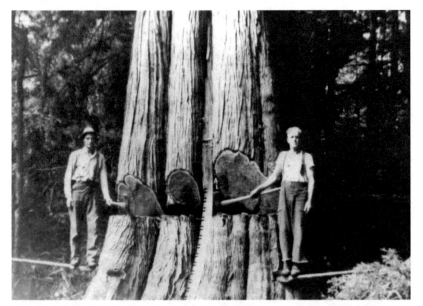

Figure 2: Grandfather and uncle on springboards, 1930s

Dad was a big raw-boned, no-nonsense type of man. Later, my brother and I said he could draw his belt for a spanking faster than Roy Rogers could draw his gun. A totally honest man, his word was his bond. That was a time when 'men were men' and 'trees were trees.' In this logging setting pets were not to be found.

My mom had her own story to tell. She was born in 1915 on the Kitsap Peninsula, a ferry ride across Puget Sound from Seattle. The economy of Kitsap County was better than Gray's Harbor's during the Depression Era, as it was not dependent on logging. It had the bustling Bremerton Naval Shipyard for employment. Money was still circulating, as one either worked in the shipyard or worked for someone who did.

Growing up in a family of twelve children, they had little space, time, or money to be spent on a pet. Mom and two of her sisters each had one blouse and skirt for school, which they traded daily to wear something different to high school. Maybe because of those hard times she certainly wanted a better life for her own children. She met my father, married, and soon moved as a young bride to the coastal logging town.

My brother was born in 1941, eight months before the Pearl Harbor attack and the beginning of World War ll. With a son, Mom wished to move away from the ocean nearer to her family. A small farm in Kitsap County was purchased. Dad commuted from our farm to the coastal logging camps. For many years Dad was a logger during the week and did double duty, catching up on the farm work on the weekends. There was always wood and hay to get in while caring for the livestock. Into this farm setting, I was born in 1944; growing up with daily chores, a strong work ethic and no sentimental feelings for a pet.

This was an anxiety ridden time in America's history. World War II was still raging. Mom told me of dreams she had of Japanese soldiers parachuting out of the sky into the field behind the house; that anxiety added to the hardships. There were huge, tethered barrage balloons everywhere in the sky to deter Japanese war planes from attacking the local naval shipyard. By the time I was old enough to appreciate the uncertainties of the war, it was over. The country was celebrating its victory. The economy was on the upswing, the dollar was almighty and we were the world center of industrial production. It was a great time and place for our own family. The hardships and anxieties were easing. Dad could work away from the home and provide comfortable support for the family. Mom was the traditional home maker, keeping the home fires burning, while caring for my brother and me.

My first actual memories of farm life were in 1948. Reminiscent of Betty MacDonald's *The Egg and I*, our farm was similar to the setting highlighted within the book and movie. A young Marine moved his city bride to a primitive farm site near Port Townsend on the Olympic Peninsula in Washington State to raise chickens in the late 1920s. There was no running water or electricity and it rained nearly the year around. Our lifestyle was similar in many respects to this quaint farm, although, we did have running water and electricity.

Many of my early memories revolved around time spent with Mom and the chickens (Fig. 3). My folks raised chickens for eggs and meat. Mom taught me to gather the eggs. They were carried down to the basement in large wire baskets. We candled them using a bright light to check for blood spots. The jumbo eggs were separated because they were worth more. When it came time to slaughter the chickens, their necks went on the chopping block - off came their heads. To this day the saying, "Running around like a chicken with its head cut off," brings back a vivid memory of life on a farm. The folks also raised calves and pigs. Milk cows completed our rural life. Raising livestock was a necessary economic pastime for our family.

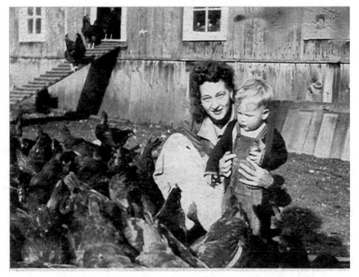

Figure 3: Mom and I feeding the chickens

In our farm setting, where did 'animals as pets' have value? Our first dog was a cocker spaniel named Penny (Fig. 4). In those days you didn't buy pets, they were either given to you or you picked up a puppy or kitten on the way out of the local feed store. Penny's value was in rounding up whatever needed rounding up, along with patrolling and protecting the farm, and with what little time was left, watching after my brother and me. Pets in our area were not kept for sentimental or companionship reasons.

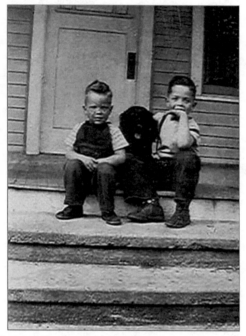

Figure 4: Penny watching after my brother and me

Cats just appeared in the barn (Fig. 5). As a group they were feral, definitely not friendly to play with, but they did keep the mice under control. The number of barn cats went up and down. When there was an unwanted litter, and there were many of them, I remember Dad putting them in a feed sack and they would just disappear. I figured they must not be worth much. Yet, a more pleasant memory with the barn cats was during milking time. They would wait patiently until a teat was turned their way. Opening their mouths in unison, whoever was doing the milking would try to fill all the mouths with one squirt.

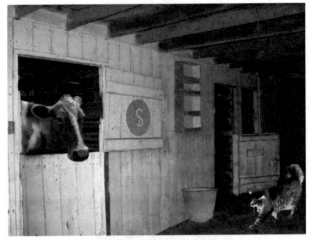
Figure 5: Feral Barn Cats

Mom fed and cared for Penny, but a dog would never be allowed inside the house. I don't remember commercial pet food ever being purchased from a store. The barn cats lived on mice and birds while Penny thrived on table scraps. I have no memory of a veterinarian coming to the farm to treat the animals. To my knowledge, we never took an animal into a veterinary office. Animals either got well on their own, were slaughtered, or simply not allowed to suffer.

As if my parents didn't have enough to do, they also planted and sold lettuce and strawberries at the local farmers' market. Money, one way or another, seemed to be at the center of most conversations or conflicts. With my dad logging away from home during the week, mom had all she could handle on the farm. Dad would come home on Friday night and frantically attempt to catch up on the ever growing and ongoing tasks. A strong memory is Dad jogging to the chicken house with two one hundred pound sacks of chicken feed, one on each shoulder. Needless to say there was not a lot of idle time.

As events would happen, an animal finally arrived on our farm without a purpose. This was not your typical pet; Blackie was a crow (Fig. 6). My brother and I were at the back of the property when a large crow suddenly appeared on the trail in front of us. I sprinted back to the house to get some bread. After feeding the crow, we were able to pick up the bird and take it home. Previously, Blackie must have been someone's pet; she could talk. She could distinctly pronounce a number of words. We taught the noisy bird to say, among other phrases, "Black crow be quiet." One day she brought me a quarter in her beak. Later that same day, she brought another quarter. I thought she had found a treasure chest. In hopes of finding the hoard of money, I followed her for several days without success. Blackie's funny antics provided several years of entertainment to the family. Then one day she just disappeared. Since she stayed outside it is likely she was taken by a hawk or coyote, so much for my first pet bird.

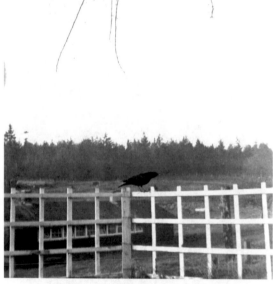

Figure 6: Blackie, our pet crow

My first 'horse' was a pig. Woof, woof, two jumps... and you were off! Being bucked off a pig in a pig pen was an interesting experience. It not only took courage to get back on the pig, but great courage to face your mom smelling like a pig pen. Mom asked me in no uncertain terms to stay off the pigs. A persistent youth, I just had to try riding a pig one more time. As luck would have it, Dad happened to see me riding that pig again. I thought here comes a spanking, but surprisingly, he calmly said, "John, stay off the pigs. They can not sweat and when they overheat they lose weight and weight is money." For the sake of protecting my bottom and our bottom line, I knew it was past time to stop riding the pigs.

My second 'horse' was a calf. This was a whole new challenging experience (Fig. 7). Straddling the calf and holding on tight, I'd circle precariously around the pasture. The calf would periodically stop to eat grass and when you wanted to move you reached back, twisted the tail and off you went. Again, Dad lectured me about riding the livestock. He said, "John, don't get too attached to that calf. It is going to be butchered next week." Well, so much for my second 'horse.' My parents finally decided that it was time I stopped riding the livestock before I broke a leg; so they bought me my first real horse.

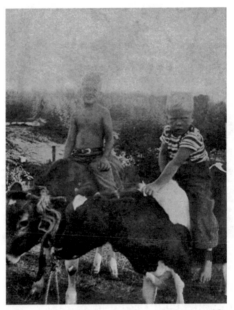

Figure 7:   My second 'horse' was a calf

Finally, an animal arrived on the farm with no economic purpose. I was eight years old and had my own horse. This was the first time I was allowed to become deeply bonded to an animal (Fig. 8). Gypsy was my responsibility and mine to ride through the pastures and trails of my childhood. With a BB gun in one hand and the reins in the other, I was off to live the life of a cowboy.

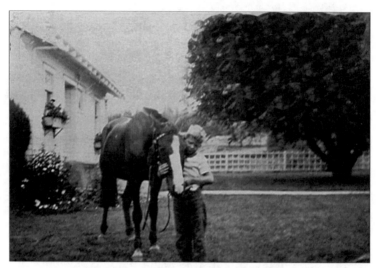

Figure 8:   Gypsy was my first real horse.

Cisco Kid was one of my many cowboy heroes (Fig. 9). At this time my parents also purchased a horse named Sugar for my brother. Together, there were logging roads to be ridden, races to be run and serious riding to be done. We would be riding for hours. It was a more trusting era for parents. The only regret I have with the time spent with Gypsy was hunting birds and squirrels; literally anything that moved in the woods was seen as fair game for target practice. Little did I imagine the reverence for life I would later acquire as a practicing veterinarian.

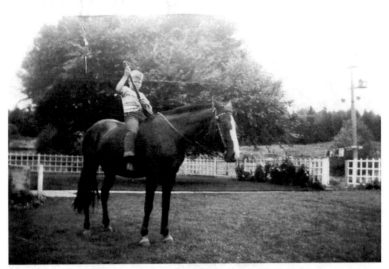

Figure 9: Gypsy and I are ready to ride.

My brother's horse, Sugar, was faster than Gypsy, but not fast enough. He wanted a really fast horse, faster than his friends' horses. Dad and my brother went to an estate sale where Thoroughbred horses were to be auctioned. They were the high bidder on a racehorse named What Do. Thrown into the deal was a goat named Nanny, who - as a stall companion - calmed What Do during her racing days (Fig. 10). What Do was a fast horse on the racetrack, but she was a really fast horse around our neighborhood. No one knew at the time that she would be the reason for my dad's next economic endeavor, as well as the motivation for my future career with animals.

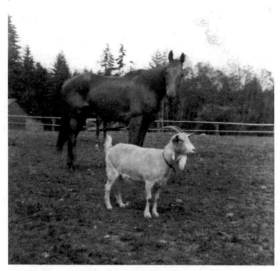

Figure 10: What Do and Nanny are stall mates.

By the mid-1950s life on the farm was changing. The chickens, pigs, calves, and cows were gone. No more planting, harvesting and selling produce. Mom was working outside the home as a meat wrapper. Dad had given up his logging commute and taken a logging job closer to home. My brother and I were involved in sports. There was more time for leisure. My life, as I had known it, was about to change. Mom decided it was time for the family to move closer to town. They found a much smaller farm only a mile from town. Leaving our childhood memories, my brother and I rode What Do and Gypsy to their new home.

Entering our adolescent years my brother and I were finding less time for riding horses. It was 1957, and I was 13 years old. Gypsy and What Do were grazing in the back pasture. Dad was getting older too. He had logged for thirty years and with the logging industry in decline it was time to leave the woods. Fortunately, he was able to gain employment with the county road department. Even then, my dad wasn't one to sit still. He always needed a project. Although neither he nor mom had any experience with the race horse industry, they decided to have What Do bred. Their intent was to raise a Thoroughbred foal

for a racing career. After careful research, What Do was bred
with a stallion related to Man o' War, and so began the wait and
anticipation for a foal. Dad shared his plan with a fellow logger,
Bill, who had recently sold his logging company. Bill liked
the idea of a race horse business, so they formed a partnership.
What started as an idea to have a single foal expanded into a
race horse breeding business. Bill would be the trainer on the
race track, while dad would oversee the breeding, foaling and
preparation of the yearlings for the track. Dad's project seemed
like a well thought out business adventure.

What Do's foaling and the subsequent events would have a
profound impact on my life. What Do went into labor in the
early morning hours. Her labor proceeded with straining and
strong abdominal contractions. Although no one in the family
had ever witnessed a foaling, we knew horses typically have a
short labor. After an hour of repeated labor efforts, we felt that
something had to be wrong. It was the first time I ever heard
Dad say, "Call the veterinarian."

Dr. King arrived shortly and did an examination. With concern
he said, "She has twin foals, but they are both dead and she can
not deliver them herself." The whole delivery was brutal and
heart-wrenching. Dad wasn't one to show his emotions, but at
this time he had to leave the barn. Dr. King flushed the mare's
uterus, instilled medication, and gave an antibiotic injection.
Then he turned to my brother and I, explaining because of the
difficult delivery What Do was very likely to develop a uterine
infection and any hope of preventing this would require daily
medical attention. He was unable to stop by each day, but a
family member would be capable of doing the treatments. By
default, I was chosen to follow through with the care. Dr. King
instructed me with what needed to be done and demonstrated
the treatments. He left the medical supplies and told me if there
were any questions to call his office. He would come to re-
examine What Do in a week's time.

After two days of treatment, What Do was not doing well. She was running a fever and had gone off her feed. We called Dr. King who performed another examination. As foretold by his previous concerns, she had developed a severe uterine infection, and in a serious tone informed the family that she may not recover. He intensified the medical treatment schedule and changed medications, so I was now treating her three times a day. To the surprise of everyone, she gradually started to improve. Later, as a complication possibly related to her uterine infection, she developed laminitis, an inflammation of the hoof. After several weeks of treatment she was back to normal.

I firmly believed it was my persistence in care and dedication to her well being that determined her recovery. This recovery was accompanied by a huge feeling of satisfaction and accomplishment. I had saved an animal's life.

Certain impressions often shape values when you are not even aware of it happening. At some moment in that old barn, I felt a calling as to my life's purpose. I would be a veterinarian.

There was a particular problem concerning my newfound passion. Mom had always wanted me to be a dentist. Without fluoride in the water, my brother and I had developed dental cavities with all the associated expenses. Those cavities and expenses motivated her desire for my future dental career. Mom had even told all our relatives that I was going to be a dentist. Feeling deeply about my new found passion, there was concern that mom wouldn't agree with my choice. Finally, I went to her and said, "Mom, I so enjoyed saving What Do, would it be O.K. if I became a veterinarian?" She looked to the left, then to the right, and after what seemed at least five minutes she said, "That would be fine." Now it was up to me.

It was at this time a special friend came into my life. My folks acquired a male boxer dog that we named Rebel (Fig. 11). Rebel and I seemed to immediately connect, maybe because I had more time to spend with him. Among my fondest memories of Rebel was telling him all my adolescent problems, as well as the hunting, exploring, and camping trips together out under the stars. It seemed his whole day would light-up when I arrived home from school; I often sat with my arm over his shoulder sharing a sandwich on the porch. Doing my chores, I always had a sidekick. At that time though, I really couldn't verbally express the feelings that I had for him. It wouldn't be until the 1960s, when the term human-pet bond crept into our vocabulary, that I understood my attachment to Rebel and the value he brought into my life.

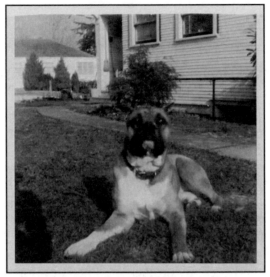

Figure 11: Rebel was my first dog.

Meanwhile, the breeding farm was coming together. We built a new ten stall barn and fenced and crossed-fenced our ten acre farm. Several mares and a stallion were purchased and the business swung into full operation. There was so much to do, but the anticipation of having a stake's winning horse on the track made work not seem like work. The mares were bred, foals delivered, yearlings broken to ride and off they went for training at the racetrack (Fig. 12). During those years, besides cleaning numerous stalls, I was involved in the veterinary care on the farm and later as a groom at the race track.

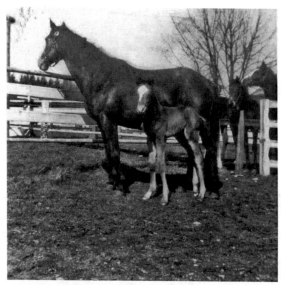

Figure 12: Mare with foal, yearlings ready to race

We had good racehorses, but never the success of a stake's
horse. After several years with our horses racing at the tracks
up and down the West Coast, the revenue from the prizes never
quite met the expense of racing. With the business reality of
horse racing more difficult than envisioned, the partnership
was eventually dissolved. Later mom was famous for saying,
"We never made any money with race horses, but we got a
veterinarian out of it!" The lesson from my parents, again, was
that an animal's value was seen purely in economic terms, but I
had experienced and felt something very different...the love of
a pet.

By my senior year in high school, I was completely focused
on becoming a veterinarian. Yet, the cost of attending a four
year college for my pre-med coursework was economically
prohibitive. A decision was made to attend our local community
college and transfer to a university after two years. Along with
a heavy class load, I worked most afternoons at a local food
supermarket. If some nights I was just too tired to complete
my studies, Mom would say, "Get to bed." Early the next
morning she would literally pull me out of bed to complete
my studies before classes began. When my work and studies

schedule challenged my motivation, mom would say, "Four or forty, John…four or forty." From previous conversations, I knew she was referring to four years of studying and getting a college degree versus forty years of working in the dangerous environment of the logging camps. Needless to say the work ethic my parents imparted was a big part in the success of my endeavors.

I completed the pre-med veterinary college admittance requirements, applied to veterinary school, did my in-person interview at the college and simply expected to be rejected. If rejected, I planned to transfer to Washington State University to improve my chances. When the letter arrived from the veterinary college, Mom simply placed it on the kitchen table. I dreaded opening the envelope and reading rejection. Yet, the first words were, "Congratulations! You have been admitted to the Washington State University College of Veterinary Medicine." The rest of the letter was a blur. Mom just nodded in approval. I was nineteen years old and would be off to veterinary college in the fall. A strong desire to help animals tempered by barn cat values and childhood experiences in a changing veterinary profession were about to collide.

Chapter Two

Box of Puppies

"I wish people would realize that animals are totally dependent on us, helpless, like children, a trust that is put upon us."

-James Herriot-

It was 1964 and the veterinary school freshman class at Washington State University was seated for orientation. Dr. Johnson, head of the Physiology Department, entered the room to present the orientation. He was older, studious in appearance with thick glasses halfway down his nose. Looking over the top of his glasses, he began to speak. "Welcome… and congratulations on your acceptance into Veterinary Medicine. You wouldn't be sitting here unless you were a good student, but from this point forward, you will experience increased academic demands made challenging by the speed and volume of material that will be presented. Look to your right, and your left, one of these students will not be here at the end of this freshman year." That statement captured my attention. He may have overestimated the attrition rate but not the academic rigor. Ultimately, six of my fifty classmates did not make it through the first year of the program.

The diversity of where and how my fellow students grew up, their personalities, levels of education, and reasons for becoming veterinarians made our class an eclectic gathering. There were five women in our class, a very high number from previous years. The profession since its inception had been viewed as too physically rigorous for women. Most students came from the western states, including Alaska. Some had already earned multiple college degrees. True to that era, many desired to be large animal practitioners and would return home to practice in a rural setting, especially students from Montana. Others envisioned being part of a mixed practice, caring for both livestock and family pets. Only a small minority planned to live in an urban setting and limit their practice to pets. For me, equine surgery was my intention. I wanted to be the veterinarian Kentucky horse owners called to save million dollar horses. It promised to be a challenging four years.

Academically, throughout my freshman year, I was doing double duty trying to catch up with my classmates who were better prepared in basic science concepts. Yet, by the sophomore year, I felt more on an academically level playing field. It is interesting to reflect that, throughout my freshman and sophomore years, I never touched a live animal. Textbooks, lectures, and labs filled each day. It wasn't until the junior year that students were allowed into the university veterinary hospital with hands-on clinical experience.

All students took small and large animal medicine and surgery. It quickly became apparent that most students had preference for one discipline over the other.

Things were changing. There were rustlings within groups of clinical professors concerning how many hours would be allotted to their courses. The amount of time needed for teaching clinical pathology and courses involving pet care came into direct conflict with the historically pre-established curriculum. One of our large animal medicine professors had his course cut from five to three hours. Maybe because he had basically used the same notes for two decades or he really believed we needed to know the historical significance of turn of the century illnesses, he informed us he would present an extra hour of his course before the normal class time. It was a memorable moment. The professor came into the classroom, uncapped a sixteen ounce bottle of RC Cola, opened a bag of peanuts, and poured them into the bottle. Then he informed us that the material from the early morning lectures would be included on his examinations. So we would all be welcome to come to class at seven am. Then he walked over to the door and closed it. Needless to say, no one was late to the extended morning hour class. The story gets embellished through the years, but it was effective: we learned livestock medicine. Later, we learned from the upper classmen this had been his morning ritual for years. At that time, my education was at least sixty percent equine, livestock, and poultry.

A dramatic shift in veterinary education was forced by the increasing value people were placing on pets. Suddenly cats were not viewed medically as small dogs, but as separate entities with their own diseases, which clients wanted addressed. Naturally, some of the students and professors dedicated to large animal medicine and surgery were a bit defensive and often viewed the emerging pet practice as something for those who didn't want to get their hands dirty. I share this not to disparage anyone, but to shed light on the impending changes in pet care that were about to redirect the economic focus of much of the veterinary profession. A new paradigm in veterinary animal care was emerging right in the middle of my studies.

Animal humane organizations were established at the turn of the century to prevent cruelty and suffering. At that time their focus was on the harsh conditions working horses were enduring on the streets of New York and Boston. Their efforts have expanded into many avenues including pet overpopulation and minimizing euthanasia. Previous to this era, during small animal surgical labs, the students anesthetized dogs, performed multiple surgeries, and then euthanized them. That was how we learned our basic surgery. Part of the evolution of this era was the development of alternative veterinary teaching methods. There was an increased awareness and concern for animal suffering and pain. Animal rights and humane movements have and will continue to elevate consciousness regarding the human-animal connection.

During this time of increasing demand for pet care, many other movements were evolving that would affect the veterinary profession. The Animal Welfare Act was passed in the fall of 1966. This law set minimal care standards for animals sold and used for experimentation. Humane and animal rights organizations were becoming increasingly active promoting animal well being. Advocates among the animal rights movement were supporting the concept that much of the information needed to benefit mankind could be acquired without animal experimentation and sacrifice.

Awareness and management of animal pain has taken monumental steps since my veterinary school years. In the 1960's, post operative animal pain was not addressed. It was a common view that pain after surgery was good because it kept the pet quiet during recovery. The many, safer pain killers of today were not available. Surgery related pain is now managed not only for compassionate and humane reasons for the animals, but to reduce patient recovery time. Monitoring pain now extends into many areas of clinical practice. It is not just a surgical issue, but improves the quality of life for a myriad of patients from those with arthritis to terminal illnesses. Pain management is a constant companion of the race horse world.

During the summer between my junior and senior year I worked for the racing commission at a thoroughbred race track near Seattle. At that time my career goal was still to be an equine practitioner with a specialty in lameness, but during that summer my job was a "pee boy." I was part of a team effort to monitor the winner of a horse race to be sure it had not been given a performance enhancing drug. After the saliva test, I would follow the race winner to the barns and collect a urine sample, seal it and return it to the commissioner's office. To further my career goal, I was also assisting one of the track veterinarians with surgeries. In his off-track veterinary facility we performed joint surgeries, primarily removing bone chips. At some point in time during this period, I became disillusioned with my long held career goal of being an equine practitioner. Career indecision filled my mind, but passion to help animals never wavered.

The summer came to an end and I returned to school for my senior year. Shortly after the beginning of the year, there was an opportunity to attend a guest lecture. The visiting lecturer started his presentation with the opinion that the veterinary profession would shortly be impacted by the proliferation of pet practices, driven by what he referred to as a human-animal bond theory. Time would prove his theory to be extremely visionary. His theory was that pet sentimentality and practical uses of this bond could dramatically change how people viewed animals. Is this why the college administration was now emphasizing pet care in our curriculum?

Pets were often considered a possession to keep or discard, or on the other extreme, a pet was considered a luxury item. There was still the age-old belief that the value of an animal was weighed against what it could earn, produce or as food on the table. This new concept that sentimentality could become a determining factor in valuing an animal seemed foreign to me, and I suspect, to many of my classmates. Yet, with the special bond I had felt with my horse Gypsy and dog Rebel combined with the increasing hiring opportunities in pet practice, I could understand the visionary wisdom of the guest lecturer's message. Yet, at that time, I could never have imagined how the increasing awareness, depth and utilization of this unique bond would manifest in so many different avenues and people's lives.

Clinical application became a significant aspect of my senior year. I was chosen to become a senior intern and live in housing provided within the veterinary teaching hospital. My main duty was assisting with small animal emergency care during the night time hours. From previous experiences, perceived career opportunities and the satisfaction I was receiving from helping pets in emergency situations, I chose small animal practice for my veterinary career path.

It was during my senior year that one needed to be serious about seeking a veterinary position. There were ten pet practitioner job offers for every student. I was twenty-three years old but looked eighteen. While taking histories and doing physical examinations, clients' perceptions were as if they were patiently waiting for someone who looked old enough to be a doctor to enter the room. Maybe it was my youthful appearance or maybe a lack of experience, but I questioned my ability to inspire client confidence and trust in caring for their beloved pet. With this mindset, I looked to find an internship at an established institution to gain more experience in small animal practice.

At the time, there were a limited number of veterinary internships. The two I was advised to apply for were offered by the Massachusetts Society for the Prevention of Cruelty to Animals; referred to as the S.P.C.A. One of the internships was in Boston at the Angell Memorial Hospital and the other in Springfield, Massachusetts at the Rowley Memorial Hospital. I was fortunate to be accepted into the program at Rowley.

The S.P.C.A. has a long history within veterinary medicine. George Angell was the founder of the Massachusetts Society for the Prevention of Cruelty to Animals. Francis Rowley, the president of the society - to honor Angell - conceived the idea of a memorial animal hospital. The construction for Angell Memorial Hospital began in 1913. In 1931 the S.P.C.A. honored Francis Rowley by establishing Rowley Memorial Animal Hospital. The S.P.C.A. Memorial Animal Hospitals would illustrate humane principles in action by providing proper pet veterinary medical and surgical treatment. I share this history because I felt honored to be chosen and given the opportunity to gain further clinical experience while supporting their mission.

On the first morning of my internship, I found myself dressed in starched white pants and jacket, pastel shirt and dark tie with a stethoscope in my pocket. This was the strictly enforced daily intern dress standard. The first client and patient that afternoon combined with an experience the following morning, would provide me with a long-term dilemma.

The client was an older gentleman with his springer spaniel, Buffy. In taking the history, besides the signs of vomiting, depression and increased urination, he wanted me to know that his wife had recently died. Together, they had loved Buffy as one would a child. I had heard this attachment level for a pet before, but what he was to tell me next was definitely new. His voice softened and he told me he felt his wife's soul had entered Buffy; allowing her to live on beyond memories. I truly felt he was sincere with his feelings. Without commenting, I examined Buffy but was unable to establish a diagnosis to explain her symptoms. Blood and urine samples were taken and submitted to the lab with a special request for immediate results. The lab results came back within an hour and they were not good. Buffy was sickened with chronic late stage kidney failure. There wasn't a good option for this diagnosis and to this day it carries an unfavorable prognosis. No time to sit and ponder; the appointment book was full.

When we got back together to review the results of the tests, I told the client the seriousness of the diagnosis. Even though I knew in my heart Buffy wasn't likely to recover, I felt my client needed time to accept the prognosis. I would do my best to improve Buffy's kidney function. I began intravenous fluids and supportive care, but Buffy's health continued to deteriorate as the day progressed. The old man sat with Buffy through out the day and into the night. I too cried, with the client, as he held Buffy while her life passed away shortly after midnight. I was physically and emotionally drained. The next day would come early with clinical responsibilities beginning at eight in the morning.

On the morning of the second day of my internship, I entered the hospital through the reception area. The receptionist had clients standing in front of her with all she could handle. She asked me for a favor as she handed me a box of newborn puppies.

"Take these abandoned puppies to the back." I carried them back and gave them to an attending assistant, informing him that they had been abandoned. As he was leaving the room with the puppies, I asked him where he was taking them. Without hesitation he announced, "They are going downstairs likely to be euthanized."

His response stopped me. Just the night before I had given my best efforts in what I believed to be a hopeless illness, consoling a client as his pet died. In contrast to that event, this morning I was a conduit to the euthanasia of a box full of healthy puppies. I could have helped these puppies, but for reasons out of my control, I was not allowed to do so.

I was learning early on in my internship that - even at a humane organization - the issues of attachment and costs would often dictate which pets got treated and which did not. The same questions now reappeared concerning my idealism for helping pets versus how they are valued: Was getting paid for services more important than a pet's life? What about the veterinarian's oath pledging to protect animal health? What is my purpose and obligations as a small animal veterinarian? Questions which echoed back to my childhood values and my experiences in veterinary school had leapt into the earliest days of my internship.

It was not long after that experience that I walked once again through the back kennel room of the hospital. Noticing a small black puppy, I paused to read the information card on the gate and discovered that the pup had been dropped off that morning and was available for adoption. The little standard poodle seemed dwarfed by the large kennel. Whether it was justification or for once just seemed to be an opportunity to do the right thing at the right time, I adopted that dog on the spot and Travis became our Massachusetts pet. He easily won the affections of my wife, becoming an important part of our new life together. My wife always joked, saying he barked with a distinct Bostonian accent.

The technical staff often lightened up the day with their antics and sense of humor. They were a close group. All had worked for the S.P.C.A. for at least twenty years, one of them for forty years. At orientation the chief-of-staff informed us that if an intern couldn't get along with the staff it would be one of us, not one of them who would go. The staff was easy to work with as long as you realized who was boss. They took great pride playing tricks on the new interns. For example, I requested an x-ray for a male German shepherd dog that had been vomiting repeatedly. After several minutes I was informed my x-ray was up, meaning ready for my interpretation.

On viewing the x-ray, there was an obvious image of a small skeleton in the middle of the abdomen. I was perplexed. With the staff looking over my shoulder, I thought out loud, "Has he swallowed an animal?" This doesn't make sense, if he had swallowed an animal the intact skeleton would be in his stomach, not the intestine. As I stood scratching my head, one of the staff members said, "Doc, it's obvious; the problem is that your male dog is pregnant." With that proclamation, the whole staff slapped hands while breaking out in gut-busting laughter. I couldn't understand what was so funny. As they were soon to tell me, the x-ray wasn't of my patient. Rather, it came from their old bag-of-tricks.

Years earlier, they had taken an x-ray of a male dog with a puppy slipped under its abdomen, creating a false image of a pregnant male dog. After the laughter at my expense subsided, they presented the x-ray that I requested. As I was to learn, these antics were a tradition and done to keep the seriousness of patient care in perspective. I came to appreciate how trying to find a humorous side of a situation could help one cope with sad cases.

Humor was everywhere if I would allow myself to step outside the seriousness of medical standards as well as some of my childhood perspectives. Many of the most humorous and fun incidences occurred when clients dressed their pets up in clothes. This was in the 1960s, when popular culture considered pet clothes a bit frivolous - albeit silly - even in the major cities or particularly in the farm towns of my childhood. For instance, on one afternoon I entered the examination room to find a yellow golden retriever sitting quietly on the table. He had a Scottish tam on his head and was wearing a Celtic plaid coat. There was a curved pipe in his mouth (Fig. 13). That in itself was memorable, but the client was identically dressed, including the pipe. The client removed his pipe and said in a Scottish brogue, "Doctor, meet my son, MacTavish." Smiling, I completed the routine appointment and as my assistant helped the patient off the table, the client said, "MacTavish, thank the good Doctor!"

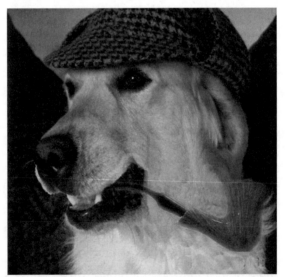

Figure 13: Meet my son, MacTavish

In another appointment, I could not help but take special notice of the pet of two elderly sisters. Their miniature schnauzer named Baby was dressed in a ballerina tutu. Without any comment, I diagnosed an ear infection and prescribed medication. In visiting with the two sisters, towards the end of the appointment, I commented that Baby's dress was quite pretty. They thanked me for the compliment and informed me that they hand-stitched all of her clothes. Since I now seemed interested, one sister asked me if I would like to see some of Baby's other clothes. I said, "That would be nice."

The next morning I was asked to come out to the reception area where the two sisters had carried in a large trunk - they opened to show dozens of different dresses and outfits they had sewn for Baby. Today, pet clothing and costumes are commonly sold in the multibillion dollar pet products industry. It would be years before I would fully understand the nature of their attachment; some pets were starting to come first, complete with a wardrobe.

Unfortunately, not all pets were so fortunate. Evelyn Stewart presented her female Persian cat, Precious, with a large abscess on her tail. Evelyn indicated Precious had been on the porch three days earlier when a stray cat attacked her. What was needed to help Precious was medically straightforward - or so I thought. An anesthetic needed to be administered, the abscess drained and flushed and a drain placed. Evelyn indicated Precious was her constant companion and ever so dear. She was sure the infection would be addressed but, because of a tight budget, she needed an estimate. Estimates are routine in a veterinary practice, so one was prepared and presented. Upon viewing the expenses she said her husband was in the car and would I mind explaining what needed to be done and go over the estimate again with him. The appointment time was up, but decisions concerning treatment consent were a necessary part of my involvement.

Eventually, Evelyn's husband entered the examination room and said "What's up?" Although ten minutes late for my next appointment, I patiently explained the abscess, its treatment and the estimate of the costs. He seemed to tense and said "Doc, it's just a cat. I'd never spend that kind of money on a cat. The cat and I have never gotten along. Anyway, don't cats have nine lives and fix themselves?" Evelyn was tearing up and

I'm now fifteen minutes late for my next appointment. I asked them to talk it over and make a decision and I'd return between appointments.

When I returned, they were not talking or looking at one another. Evelyn said it was about the money. I told her the office manager may be able to arrange credit. The possibility of credit did not elicit any response from the husband with arms tightly folded. Evelyn said they would take Precious home and call me in the morning. No phone call ever came. It seemed other values may have won out over Evelyn's emotional attachment for Precious.

I would see many variations to this money-emotion dilemma over the coming decades, which I would need to sort out within myself and also develop tools of compassion to aid clients in these difficult moments. In the years that followed—with my own practice—I would have the freedom and compassionate flexibility necessary to find viable options for almost any clinical situation.

At this time, one set of clinical challenges that lacked viable options were serious pet eye problems. A serious eye problem is painful for the pet and an emotional event for the owner. At Rowley, a premier pet care facility, I had seen too many pets lose an eye. In the late 1960s, widespread knowledge, diagnostics or care for acute animal eye disease was limited within the veterinary profession. When a pet was presented with sudden onset ocular pain it was most often treated with an eye ointment and if that failed the eye was removed. Given the advancements in human ophthalmology, I felt there must be better options for treating serious animal eye conditions beyond ointments or removal of the eye. Animal care specialization was still in its early stages.

I learned that Ohio State University had an advanced program in animal ophthalmology. Since I was approaching the end of my internship in Massachusetts, I applied for the ophthalmology position and was accepted into the program. Because of my acceptance, my wife and I tightly packed all our possessions in our Volkswagen bug. With our standard poodle Travis and our parakeet Petie, we headed west for Columbus, Ohio.

My goal, while at the university's ophthalmic program, was to acquire advanced knowledge and skills to help pets - including horses - with serious ocular conditions. As I would soon come to discover, the program had broader designs than just clinical animal ophthalmology. Comparative ophthalmic knowledge was acquired through time spent in classes held at both the university's human medical hospital and the university's veterinary hospital. I learned instrumentation skills needed for diagnostics with the residents in the human ophthalmology program. At the veterinary college my responsibilities included teaching classes and helping to make research contributions, while carrying a clinical case load. All of this while taking graduate level classes at the graduate school. At the time, there was no formalized residency program for a veterinary ophthalmologist; the Board in this specialty did not come into being for three more years.

The program I was attending was invigorating, challenging and at times a bit overwhelming. The richness of my studies only reinforced my desire for practical clinical applications. Later, the desire by others to institutionalize advanced skills and knowledge would lead to the formation of specialty boards. Their formation would not have occurred without the evolving importance of pets.

The outstanding professors and learning opportunity provided by Ohio State University gave me the knowledge and skills I was seeking to be able to deliver a higher degree of eye care. I probably still looked too young to be a doctor, but my veterinary school education, my internship and specialty training gave me the confidence to know I was ready to help clients and their pets. My wife and I, along with our pets tightly packed in our small Volkswagen bug, headed west again—but this time without a job or place to stay.

Chapter Three

Glasses on Dogs

"It often happens that a man is more humanely related to a cat or dog than to any human being."

-Henry David Thoreau-

During my student days, it was said, private practice was where one found 'real' veterinarians. In a historical perspective, 'real' veterinarians were those rugged individuals who performed physically challenging procedures, often in harsh weather conditions, conserving livestock resources. If a veterinarian was defined by this environment, I was in serious trouble. My entrance into private practice was as an associate at a small animal hospital in Tacoma, Washington. The practice was located in a modern brick building designed exclusively for pet care.

My ability to care for complicated eye problems became known within the local veterinarian community. I started receiving a number of eye referrals. This, along with our growing general practice, created busy days and long nights. Meeting the medical needs of pets, as well as understanding the special considerations of the owner, made for challenging days; human affection for pets manifests itself in a variety of ways. Needless to say, there were many memorable clients and patients in those early practice days.

Most clients actively participate in choosing their own pet, but other's pets may arrive in unusual ways. Edna Jones' two young Chinese Shar-Pei dogs were referred to me with corneal ulcers. Their names were Rip and Van. I commented on the uniqueness of their names, interested in hearing the story of how they happened to come by them. She willingly explained that their names were related to the extensive number of wrinkles covering their bodies, a distinctive feature of the breed. Perplexed, I still didn't grasp the connection. Edna did a little eye rolling, and said expectantly, "Don't you get it, Doctor? Remember Washington Irving's short story about Rip Van Winkle!" Ah, of course, with just a little play on words we now have the suitable names Rip Wrinkle and Van Wrinkle. I finally understood the gist of the names. The two pups had been an unexpected Christmas present from her husband. As she corralled them into the exam room, she said with dramatic emphasis, "My husband thought I needed them! He bought them from the Nieman Marcus Catalogue as one of their unique gifts of the year. He paid over five thousand dollars! What on earth was he thinking?" Assuming this was a rhetorical question, I refrained from answering with none other than a smile. Shar-pei's with their novel wrinkled appearance and infectious personalities were a rarity as pets in the 1970s, only later to become quite popular.

Unfortunately, many in the breed had a genetically induced eyelid condition called entropion. This condition has one or both of the eyelids turning inward, rubbing on the cornea and often creating an ulcer. Unfortunately, on examination, Rip and Van proved to have corneal ulcers and both needed corrective surgery; not an inexpensive proposition. Shar-pei's have extra fluid in their skin tissues causing puffiness within the tissue around the eyes. That unique feature of the breed makes the surgery more difficult.

The procedure went well and our wrinkled patients were ready to go home the following day, attired in their plastic Elizabethan cone-shaped collars. On picking up her pets at discharge time,

Mrs. Jones simply looked at her two bizarrely dressed wrinkled pups and said with a sigh, "I wonder what novel idea he will have for me next Christmas!"

Memorable eye referrals were certainly not limited to traditional pets. Sweet Pea was a large python, measuring over six feet. The client, Sheila Kelly, was quite a lovely young lady, but tearfully in distress at the time of the exam. In taking the patient history, it was noted that Sweet Pea was an essential element in Ms. Kelly's exotic dance routine at the local men's club. Originally, the pet had been inherited from her brother. Being a cherished family pet for many years, Sweet Pea was more than just a professional business partner. She served a dual role in the client's life – pet and performer. Recently, to the dismay of her owner, Sweet Pea seemed to have gone blind. Ms. Kelly emphatically stated, "Sweet Pea needs her eyesight to perform!"

To lend additional perspective to this unusual case, since childhood I have had a phobia about snakes. As children growing up on the farm, my brother seemed to delight in putting a garter snake down the back of my shirt. Until this day, when I encounter a snake, I still feel a slither down my backbone.

Knowing my trepidation about snakes, my little ninety pound technician bravely reached into that large cardboard box sitting on the floor and pulled out the huge head of Sweet Pea. The rest of the snake just kept coming. Soon all six feet were accounted for on the exam table, and now it was my turn. Sweet Pea obviously had been handled before and was, all considered, a very cooperative patient. Without even using instrumentation, it was obvious she was blind. Her eyes stood out like two bluish-white marbles. Putting on a head loop for magnification and using a bright light, I cautiously moved in for a closer examination. I now was eye to eye with my childhood nemesis. My oath to protect animal health was being tested. I knew immediately the cause of her blindness; it was obvious by the appearance of the eyes. Sweet Pea was afflicted with a condition that goes by the name "retained eye cups", or more technically, "retained spectacles".

Snakes do have spectacles. Since they don't have eyelids, the spectacles serve as a protective surface over the cornea and may be thought of as similar to a contact lens. This corneal covering is made up of two clear layers. The outer layer normally will slough when the snake sheds its skin. When it doesn't slough, it turns opaque and is retained over the cornea. Most commonly the reason that a portion of the spectacle is retained is because of low household humidity.

I knew what to do about the condition and explained it thoroughly to the client. Artificial tears would be applied to the dried out surfaces of the eyes until they were well-hydrated. Then I would gently separate the outer layer from the inner layer of the retained spectacle. More specifically, I would use the flat end of a toothpick, to ease the outer layer off the python's cornea. Any forceful peeling would very likely damage the underlying corneal structure and potentially lead to permanent blindness. Fortunately, without requiring an overzealous effort, the retained spectacles were removed without incident. After surgery I instilled antibiotic ointment in both of Sweet Pea's eyes and, thank goodness, she didn't have to stay the night. As Sweet Pea and the client drove out of the parking lot, a thought entered my mind: a pet once considered bizarre is now part of an everyday veterinary practice.

Most medical conditions are usually straightforward to treat compared to the issue of pet behavioral disorders. When behavioral problems arise, they can threaten the human-pet bond. It is important to offer clients treatment options. Many of these options for behavioral disorders were not available in the 1970's when I first met Jake and his owner.

Jake was a one year old male boxer that Susan Olsen had rescued from the adoption center. When she first acquired Jake, she brought him into the clinic for a general examination, an update to his vaccinations, and any preventative care needs.

He appeared to be a strong, healthy, young dog and seemed very content with his new owner. A few months later, Jake was brought back into the clinic for a behavioral concern. On taking his history, Miss Olsen indicated that she had just about reached her wit's end. She said, "He's destroying the house! When he's home alone: he barks incessantly, digs holes in the doors and pulls curtains off the windows. Yesterday, he chewed a hole down to the springs in my new leather couch." She continued, "He's content when I'm home; just follows me around." She was considering returning Jake to the adoption center, but it would break her heart. However, she felt she may have no other option. Jake's behavior was out of control.

In the early 1970s, the veterinary profession's knowledge of abnormal animal behavior was very limited. At the time, there wasn't a name to describe Jake's behavior other than 'bad doggie.' All I could do was sympathize with Miss Olsen's dilemma. Trying to ease the situation, I prescribed some tranquilizers just as I would for a pet reacting strongly to a Fourth of July fireworks display. Then I remembered some colleagues talking about a retired 'people' psychologist who had some success dealing with behavioral issues in pets. I rediscovered his name and passed it on to the client as someone who might be able to help her deal with Jake's situation. This was definitely not a veterinary medical issue.

Referring a client and her pet to a psychologist was definitely ahead of the times. Today, veterinarians do have a name for this specific behavioral abnormality. It is referred to as separation anxiety, is quite common, and appears in various degrees. Difficult patients can now be referred to a veterinary behaviorist, who is the psychiatrist of our profession. As a general principal, punishment is rarely effective in dealing with a pet's behavior disorder and often times will make a situation worse. Before referring a pet to an animal behaviorist, medical concerns need to be ruled out as the cause for the abnormal behavior. Medication, environmental changes and behavior modification are today's tools of choice for pet behavior disorders.

Later, Miss Olsen related to me that, although there had been improvements in Jake's behavior, it was still somewhat problematic. Changes had been made in the boxer's physical environment whenever he was left home alone. The psychologist had also given her some behavioral modification techniques that definitely seemed to help the situation. No medications for this behavioral disorder were prescribed because they were not available at this time. The client was happy to report that she was able to keep her pal, Jake.

Another behavioral disorder commonly referred is associated with old dog cognitive dysfunction, a model for Alzheimer's in man. Behavioral disorders are not limited to dogs, a variety of species are referred to animal behaviorists. Cats have their behavioral issues, often seen as inappropriate soiling inside the home. One of the most common bird behavioral problems is 'feather pulling.' Behavioral issues can place stress on a client's relationship with their pet.

Whenever the human-pet bond is strained or threatened, the veterinary profession must present viable options for the pet owner: being flexible in meeting the needs of the pet and the client.

Often it is difficult to discern a client's special considerations concerning their pet during an examination. Sophia, a fawn Chihuahua, was referred to me for blindness. At the beginning of the history, Janet Davis indicated Sophia had come to her as a puppy. Now her beloved pet had reached the ripe old age of nineteen years. On examination, it was apparent Sophia's blindness was caused by cataracts. With the diagnosis given, the client's discussion centered around what could be done medically or surgically to possibly restore Sophia's eyesight.

Cataract surgery in the 1970s was possible, but a successful result was far from assured and returned only partial vision. Today, the technique of cataract surgery is less invasive and includes a lens implant within the eye, providing a much better visual outcome. So even if Sophia's cataract surgery was successful, she would have only limited visual improvement. I felt the patient was too old for surgery and was truly hesitant to recommend it. After fully informing Mrs. Davis of my concerns, she only asked, "When can you do the surgery?" Suspecting I had not explained the medical concerns clearly or maybe she didn't understand the issues which heavily weighed against her pet having surgery at nineteen years of age, I repeated myself. Again, she said, "I do understand, but I still want Sophia to have the surgery."

There are times when a veterinarian needs to step back from the clinical aspects of a particular case in order to fully understand the client's considerations. Experience told me as long as the cataracts were not painful, Sophia would continue to adjust to her blindness. I needed to hear the reasons as to why it was so important to have the cataracts addressed. The client's eyes welled-up as she explained, "Sophia has been such a special part of my life and seen me through some very difficult times. I would like to do this surgery for her as a tiny payback for what she has given me." Then she added, "After all, my grandmother had cataract surgery when she was quite old." Understanding the client's perspective, I spent some time reviewing the blood work and urine tests that had been sent with the referral case file, finding the numbers to be within normal bounds. All signs indicated little Sophia would probably tolerate the anesthetic just fine and the procedure performed would be no different than that done on a younger dog. After reviewing the limitations of the surgery once again with the owner, I consented to remove the cataracts.

Surgery went well and was successful with partial vision restored. The little Chihuahua was now able to avoid objects in her path: no more getting lost in the house or bumping into table legs. The client was delighted with the results and I too was pleased, as well as relieved the surgery had gone well. We had done all that was possible for Sophia.

I was coming to realize that each client's considerations need to be part of the decisions making process, not just based entirely on medical facts and prognosis. Ms. Davis' affection for her pet had enhanced the little dog's quality of life, and it was only in the 1970s. I couldn't help but think, what if there were post-cataract surgery corrective lenses to completely restore vision back to normal?

Sophia, Jake, Sweet Pea, the Van Wrinkles, and countless other pets during our time in Tacoma had given me the confidence to believe I could manage diverse cases of a small animal private practice on my own. It was time to return to my home town and start my own practice. My wife, Patty, and I leased a small vacant church, remodeled it, borrowed money for equipment, and enthusiastically opened our own veterinary clinic in Bremerton, Washington (Fig. 14). Later, my mother-in-law would comment that we looked like two kids opening a lemonade stand. It was too late in the year to get our clinic listed in the phone book, so we advertised elsewhere and depended on word of mouth to let the community know we were open for business. Needless to say, it probably helped that I was a hometown boy returning to the area. It was an exciting day when the second phone line rang and Patty, who was also my receptionist, had to put the first line on hold.

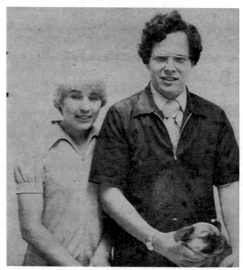

Figure 14: My wife and I open our clinic.

One of our early patients went by the name of Momma Dog. This large mixed breed dog was brought in by my friend, Linda Peters. During a routine examination and vaccination appointment, Linda voiced a concern that would have otherwise unforeseen implications for my beginning veterinary practice.

Momma Dog could not ride in the car without her head sticking out the back seat window. If the window wasn't open, she would become very anxious and create a potential driving hazard. Linda also worried about eye injuries to her pet. I reassured her even though it might be possible I had never actually seen or heard of an eye injury occurring from this situation. The best advice I could give her was to allow Momma Dog's head to be out the window because of the driving safety issue, but keep the window at least half way up to prevent her from jumping out.

A few weeks later, there was an advertisement for dog protective eyewear in a veterinary magazine. The eye wear had sturdy large frames, which gave me an interesting idea. Would it be possible to use this type of frame to put corrective lenses in front of the eyes of my cataract patients? In early medical days, people who had cataracts removed usually were fitted with glasses with corrective lenses after the surgery. Why not for dogs?

On a whim, I ordered a pair and soon received the frames in the mail. However, this provided another dilemma. If I was to put lenses in the frames, how could the strength of each lens be determined for a particular dog's vision? Calling an optometrist friend, I inquired how eye doctors knew the strength of a lens needed to use on a child. He told me it would be possible to use a refractometer to determine the best corrective lenses, even on a dog (Fig. 15). The idea of putting corrective glasses on a dog after cataract surgery was exciting.

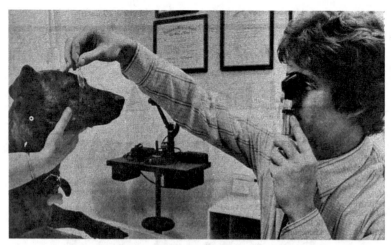

Figure 15: Optometrist refraction test on Momma Dog

A few days later, while visiting with a client during an appointment, I mentioned in casual conversation my idea of putting glasses on dogs. It just happened that the client was a reporter for our local newspaper. She became fascinated with the idea and asked me if she could take a picture of the glasses on a dog.

Momma Dog was the perfect fit for the new frames. The bespectacled dog's image was taken, along with a picture depicting an optometrist performing refraction on Momma Dog's eyes. We had quite a lot of fun with this, but the reality of actually putting glasses on a dog was still an idea in the early stages. The picture of Momma Dog and the optometrist was highlighted in our local newspaper. To my surprise, the national media quickly picked up on the article. Stories of a veterinarian and an optometrist putting glasses on a dog went nationwide. A late night TV show - filmed in California – called, inviting me to talk on their show about dogs wearing prescriptive glasses. Then, a relative of mine from the East Coast sent a clipping showing that Ripley's Believe It Or Not had done a story (Fig. 16). What had started as an idea of fitting a pet with frames and determining how to choose corrective lenses following cataract surgery had ballooned into a story that was stretched at best. I declined all TV appearances and took a low profile on the whole subject, but it was fun nonetheless!

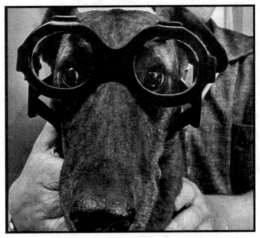

Figure 16a: Bespectacled Mamma Dog

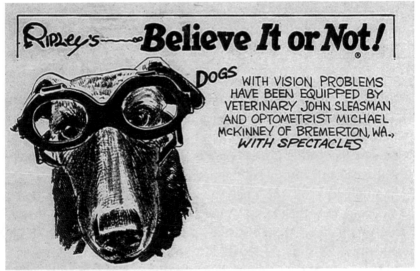

Figure 16b: *Ripley's Believe It or Not* ®

It was many years later that 'Doggles' became quite popular. This eyewear for pets expanded into fashion items, sunglasses, and protective eyewear for military dogs in the dust of the Afghanistan desert, and yes…now includes the option of prescription lenses. The use for pet eyewear continues to expand. I am sure at the time we were fitting Momma Dog, my father would have thought, "Glasses on dogs? Beyond silly!"

Dogs wearing eyewear and clothing is only one visual representation of pet attachment I have seen during my practicing years. Human affection for pets continues to manifest itself in an endless variety of ways.

Schatzie I, II, and III had been my patients over a thirty year period. All three were female red miniature dachshunds, commonly known as doxies. When Schatzie I died, they acquired Schatzie II. After she passed away, along came Schatzie III. The name Schatzie, meaning love or dear in German, is a perfect name to characterize the Millers' family feelings for their beloved pets. Since the first day of Schatzie I's life, Mrs. Miller kept a daily diary of her pet's activities. She continued the diary for all three of her Schatzies. The diary recorded each pet's daily activities, food, medications, and antics. She also wanted me to know that she had recorded every appointment's conversation we had over the past thirty years. Startled, I asked, "Every conversation?" At which point she expanded, "All preventative care, diagnoses, treatments, and follow ups." I was somewhere between fascinated and speechless.

Not having any children of their own in their lives, their pets were truly viewed as their children. When they entered the clinic for an appointment, they would always want to know all of the details, presumably for the diary. Their appointments would always run over-time, causing havoc in my busy schedule. Visiting and diagnosing simultaneously can often be a challenge, but we still managed to have many laughs together. The Millers have since passed away, but the memories of their friendship and genuine care for their Schatzies is not forgotten. The handwritten diaries are heart-warming memoirs demonstrating a special love for three special pets.

Before our three boys blessed our family life, we added our second standard poodle, Stacy. So now my immediate family had two standard poodles, as well as Petie the parakeet. I understood how clients could think of their pets as children.

It was Christmas Eve when the phone rang. My answering service had received a call concerning a cat that had been hit by a car and was having great difficulty breathing. When I called the client, the frantic voice of the lady pleaded that I see her beloved pet. She could not reach her regular veterinarian on the holiday, but she knew where my hospital was located and could bring her cat to me. My wife Patty and I headed out to meet the client at the clinic.

Arriving at the hospital, the client was holding her cat in her arms as she waited at the front door. Forgoing the normal paperwork, we quickly ushered the distraught client and her cat into the first examination room. The client indicated that she and her cat, named Fancy, lived alone and she truly thought of her cat as the light of her life. Fancy was in critical condition. I requested x-rays and the client consented. The x-rays showed the intestines within the chest were compressing the lungs which explained the cat's extreme difficulty in breathing. With a diagnosis of a ruptured diaphragm, surgery would be required and would need to be done that night to save her pet's life. Surgery on Christmas Eve was not my plan for the evening, but in those days there wasn't an emergency hospital in the county, so there really were no other viable options. The client wanted me to do the surgery and save her 'child,' an uncommon sentiment in our area. She asked what were Fancy's chances and the costs. I told her the prognosis was very guarded and the cost would run three to five hundred dollars. In those days of veterinary medicine, issues related to payment were pretty informal, especially in the middle of the night. Fancy's owner indicated she was financially stressed until her next paycheck. I explained that half the estimate could be paid and the clinic could bill her for the balance or she always had the option of not letting Fancy suffer. She knew what that meant and broke down into heavy sobbing. With feelings of compassion and

professional obligation, I told the client I would do the surgery
for twenty five dollars and wished her a Merry Christmas. The
new client wrote out a check and left to await my phone call
after the surgery.

To make a long story short, Fancy had a successful surgery.
That night she recovered from surgery next to our bed at home
and was discharged from the hospital on Christmas Day. Many
aspects of pet veterinary care certainly have changed since the
decade of the 1970s. Oh, did I mention the check bounced?

Of the many challenging emergency calls, one in particular
comes to mind. I call the case 'the sink full of puppies.' It was
after midnight when the phone rang. The answering service
had a call from a client with a dog who couldn't give birth.
Calling the client, Miss Cleveland indicated her St. Bernard,
Brandy, had been in unproductive labor for several hours.
She asked if I could meet her at the hospital and help with the
delivery. In those days every veterinarian was on his own when
it came to emergencies. My nighttime helper, my wife, was
out of town for the weekend, which would make any surgery
difficult. If there was a C-section needed, I would have to fly
solo. Greeting the client in the parking lot, I marveled at the size
of a late stage pregnant St. Bernard. During the examination,
I determined there were no puppies in the pelvic canal. Given
the length of time she had been in labor, a decision was made
to strengthen the labor contractions with a hormone. The
labor effort increased—but still no puppies. The only option
left was a C-section. It was two o'clock in the morning: there
was one veterinarian, a pregnant one hundred and thirty pound
St. Bernard, and a novice, queasy client. I had done many
C-sections, but never under these conditions. Turning to the
client, I said, "Our only option is a C-section, and if I'm to do
this, I'll need your help." She said she had never been around
surgery and was afraid she would faint at the sight of blood. I
thought, "Oh, great….I'm pretty much on my own." So I asked
her to help me lift Brandy on the surgery table and then hold
a vein so I could induce anesthetic. Then I needed her to hold

Brandy's mouth open so I could pass a tube down the windpipe. The rest I could do on my own. Miss Cleveland—with hand over her mouth—headed for the reception area to wait.

Thinking through the surgery, I realized I wasn't going to have someone to hand the puppies to after removing them from the uterus. Looking around I realized my only option was to warm the large surgical sink in preparation. I would place each puppy into the warm area after removing the birth sac. I would need to complete the surgery before I could attend to them.

On entering the abdomen, both horns of the uterus were huge. I needed to remove the puppies without bringing the uterus to the outside for fear of tearing a vessel--and so I started. Multiple uterine incisions were required. Each puppy was removed and placed in the warm sink. One after another, they just kept coming. Finally, there was an even dozen pups in the sink. Even for a St. Bernard, that was a large litter. Closing the multiple uterine incisions, the abdominal wall and the skin took over an hour. During that time, my mind kept turning to the sink full of puppies. Finally, popping off the surgical gloves and checking on Brandy, I turned my full attention to the puppies. They seemed to fill the sink. To my delight, after putting a tie on each umbilical cord and removing the membranes, all the puppies were talking and moving. At that point I involved a delighted client in rubbing and drying the newborns. We stayed up until sunrise, wakening Brandy from anesthesia and encouraging the puppies to "take turns" to nurse, as there were only ten spigots. Everyone was exhausted, including Brandy, but there was something special about that night. I had brought twelve much wanted puppies into the world and helped an appreciative client. Those were the days!

A handwritten note often provides a clear articulation of a client's love for a pet. It is curious to note that many of the nicest thank-you notes I've received as a veterinarian have been after a pet's euthanasia. I'm not sure why this is so, but feel it must be tied to the intensity of the moment and the compassion of the caregivers. Clients with aging pets often ask me when is the right time to put them to sleep. The same question often arises when a pet is faced with a terminal illness. My best answer is to assure them they will know when the time comes. Often these are patients who have had regular veterinary care over the years, but are now faced with a difficult situation. Euthanasia never gets easier.

To illustrate, I remember a case that started out with the phone ringing at three o'clock in the morning. As an on call veterinarian, good news never comes at this hour. I recognized the voice as my close friend, Paul Hinton. He was sorry to call at this hour, but he really needed my help. He said, "Darth's time has come." Darth Vader was a very old black Labrador retriever who was on pain medication and symptomatic treatment for terminal cancer. Paul asked me if I could possibly come to the house at this hour. His children were home from college and would be leaving early in the morning. Yet, it was so very important to all of the family to be present at the end of their old pet's life. This I could do for them. After stopping at the hospital to get the necessary supplies, I headed out to Paul's home.

Paul met me at the door, thanked me for coming and led me to the living room. The family was sitting in a circle around their old Lab who was lying on his mattress in the middle of the room. The whole family was holding hands and many tears had already been shed. Darth had been a wonderful friend and companion during their childhood years, filling them all with so many good memories. Yet, they knew their pet's time had come. There are never any good words at a time like this, so I just tried to reassure them, saying, "Let's do Darth a last favor and not let him suffer." Their old Lab went to sleep peacefully, surrounded by the whole family. As I said earlier, it never gets easier. I carried Darth to my car and headed back to the hospital. It seemed only fitting that the sun was just starting to rise, in honor of this beautiful dog.

There is much sadness and many times when deep compassion is needed in a veterinary practice, but there is also much joy. One day, there entered a new client that my receptionist had dubbed 'the purple lady.' My receptionist, who happened to be a close neighbor of the client, went on to explain. The purple lady had a purple house, a purple mailbox and a purple car. As she entered the animal hospital, the stately lady was dressed entirely in purple. Not only that, she carried her white miniature poodle dressed in a purple coat, a purple ribbon in her hair and purple painted toenails. After discussing her pet's medical concerns, I found it easy to overlook her eccentricity, as she was a delightful lady and a well-informed client, who just happened to like the color purple. She was one of those clients I always looked forward to seeing again at the next appointment. Over the years I've learned to expect surprises and assume nothing.

Pets seem to foster behaviors in humans that others might consider eccentric. Margaret Eddy was an elderly English lady who lived alone with fifteen Pekingese. As I learned later, her deceased husband had been a timber baron and left her without any financial concerns. This is at least part of the reason why Mrs. Eddy could be an excellent owner to so many dogs. In our role as veterinarians, our professional association has us on the lookout for pet hoarding abuse. This term is used to describe a person who reproduces pets continually and often has large numbers of uncared for animals living within the home. A large number of dogs in one home could potentially be an example. Pet hoarding abuse needs to be reported to the local humane society.

Although very likely considered an eccentric, Mrs. Eddy was not a pet hoarder. She simply had no other family, so her dogs became her immediate family. Most were spayed or neutered and appeared very well cared for by the owner. Occasionally there would appear a litter of new puppies, but it was always a planned event. She knew each of the fifteen dogs by name and treated them as individuals. All were provided excellent medical attention. While caring for her fifteen pets, we became good friends. She seemed to enjoy sharing her life stories

with me and often called for veterinary services during those
more expensive emergency hours, perhaps she wished to have
more time to talk. Mrs. Eddy was highly educated and had
even at one time performed as a dancer with a ballet company,
but most importantly, she loved her little dogs. If the fifteen
little Pekingese could have talked, I believe they would have
expounded on their good fortune in life.

Cats, with their unique personalities, make some of the most
intriguing pets. My pet cat was Emily, the free-roaming hospital
cat (Fig. 17). She seemed to own the place and greeted the
clients as they entered the hospital. My wife being allergic to
cats, in fact, horses too, we were not able to have Emily at our
home.

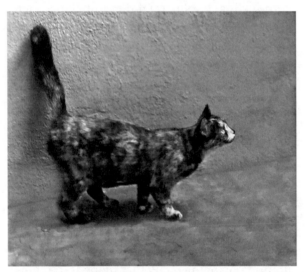

Figure 17: Emily, my cat

Usually, a woman will bring the family cat into the hospital,
but when a man alone brings his cat in to me, I expect the cat to
be cherished. A particular impromptu meeting comes to mind,
when Bill Letz with his black and white male cat, fittingly
named Tuxedo, raced into the hospital right at closing time. He
hadn't made an appointment, but was extremely anxious about
his pet. Mr. Letz and Tuxedo lived alone. He first reported
to me that in the morning his pet seemed to be fine. Arriving
home from work, Tuxedo was found yowling in his litter box.

Straining, the cat could not produce any urine. My first concern was for Tuxedo's discomfort. I must admit, my second thought was here was another night of a missed dinner. By the history alone, I knew it was likely that Tuxedo had a urinary blockage. Tens of thousands of male cats had died from urinary blockages during the 1960s and 1970s. These cats either died outright from the blockage or were put to sleep after multiple blockage recurrences. Tuxedo was in a critical condition.

At this time, the underlying cause of urinary tract blockage was unknown. It was believed that a low phosphate or ash diet, along with urinary acidifiers, prevented many recurrences. I had observed cats that lived outside and ate mice and other prey did not develop urinary blockages. Eventually, researchers would determine that commercial diet imbalances led to the plug formation. With these findings, commercial cat food manufacturers modified their foods, which greatly reduced the occurrences of urinary blockages. Even though the incidents are greatly reduced, they can still occur today. As a side note, it has been my experience that today's blockages are more difficult to unblock, have a higher incidence of recurrence, and more frequently need corrective surgery.

The typical 'blocked' cat emergency entailed a client calling to say her male cat was going to the litter box repeatedly, straining without urine production and yowling as if in distress. These were cats with early onset urinary blockages. Countless numbers of cats, as cats often do with serious illnesses, just disappeared to die of uremic poisoning. Cats that made it to the hospital were given a general anesthetic, had the gritty, crystal-filled plug flushed from their urethra, and a catheter placed into the bladder. After two to three days in the hospital, the catheter was removed. Many urinated well after this and went home with a urine acidifier and a low ash diet. While most didn't re-obstruct, some did. In Tuxedo's case, he re-obstructed three times. My rule was, three times a loser... surgery was necessary.

While at Ohio State University, I had observed a surgery that was so new that it was still in clinical trials and hadn't yet been published. The procedure was to become known as a feline urethrostomy. After surgery, the male cat would have outside 'plumbing' which resembled that of a female cat. The urethrostomy made the diameter of the urethra larger and shortened the distance from the bladder to the outside. With this accomplished the obstructing crystal-filled plugs could pass freely. Performing a feline urethrostomy was to become, and still is, the surgery of choice for repeat male cat urinary blockages. In a small animal practice, it was not unusual to consistently have a blocked cat in the hospital. I found myself frequently performing urethrostomy surgeries. After only a few years, I had done well over a hundred urethrostomies. Now it was Tuxedo's time.

Tuxedo joined the male club of rearranged external plumbing. After dealing with Mr. Letz and his pet, I realized that each of these male cats and their owners belonged to a pretty special group. Each cat seemed exceptionally gentle, and the clients were so committed to their pets. Maybe because of the anxiety of this particular condition or maybe because I had spent so much time with them, they were a unique group. So, I had an idea. Why not bring all the clients together whose cat had to have the surgery? We'd have an urethrostomy party to celebrate their pets' good health. Formal invitations were sent in the mail and on a Sunday afternoon, twenty eight cats and clients arrived at the door. As you can image, twenty eight male cats loose in the reception area created its own dynamics (Fig.18). Surprisingly, the boys all got along quite well, though admittedly a few had to have time out in the kennel room before they were able to return to the party. The menu included a low ash entrée for the cats, while clients had cake and beverages. It was a special celebration for a special group of pets and clients.

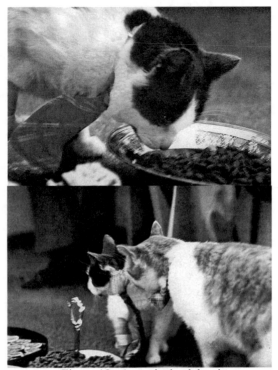

Figure 18: A surgical celebration

The diversity of cases that entered the doors our private small animal practice demanded clinical astuteness, sensitivity to people's emotions, and flexibility to family budget. These cases provide some context for the multidimensional complexities and values of the modern day human-pet bond. This bond at its best is a delightful, mutually beneficial and non-judgmental special friendship. It doesn't matter the age of the pet, the number of pets in a household, or even the type of pet, exotic or not. The difficult end of life issue only seems to make the connection even more poignant. When the bond is threatened - emotions, cost and treatment options can be in conflict, especially in a challenging economy. Most pets are thought of as part of the family today, and some even take on a childlike importance. Others may take on an almost spiritual role as a connection to a lost soul mate. The challenge for a veterinarian is meeting the needs of the pet, listening to the client's considerations, and doing everything possible to weave through the complexities of the human-pet relationship for a successful outcome.

It was the mid-70s and our little converted church was bursting at the seams. There were simply too many patients and not enough room. A new graduate from the veterinary school, Dr. Doug O'Donnell, joined my practice. He, too, was a local boy. With his involvement in the equine community, he wanted to do a mixed small animal and large animal practice. As this decade moved along, we added a third veterinarian to our practice with the necessary support staff. We had truly outgrown our existing facility. Purchasing land north of town, we built a state-of-the-art small animal hospital that could serve the ever-developing needs of our clientele. With the clinic's expansion and the growing importance of pets in society, we entered a new chapter in practice evolution with resulting improved care for pets in our community. We did it all. The joy of serving the human-pet bond was about to soar.

Chapter Four

Wolves, Seals, and Chimpanzees

"Until he extends the circle of compassion to all living things, man will not himself find peace."

- Dr. Albert Schweitzer -

Little could I have known—with the opening of the new hospital—the joy I would discover each new day in practice. Our second facility was laid out as a state-of-the-art veterinary hospital from the first stroke of the designer's pen, not having to make-do with a remodeled facility was liberating. We had the space to create specified exam rooms, pharmacy, treatment room, and surgery suites; as well as a separate isolation ward for handling infectious diseases, all with its own ventilation system and filled with the newest equipment. Yes, a new veterinary facility straight from the minds of my partner, Dr. O'Donnell, and myself. Entering the door each morning was a joy for our staff and clients... and, hopefully, to the pets as well, although they might have preferred the adjoining outdoor pet park centered by a red fire hydrant (Fig. 19).

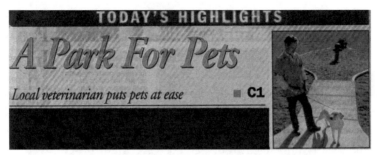

Figure 19: Hospital Pet Park with fire hydrant

This idealistic veterinary environment was energizing to our young staff, but it was more than having the 'perfect' setting that made the 1980s such a joyous time in the life of a veterinarian. This was the golden time of veterinary medicine; the end of the James Herriot era. There was a sense of community and being an active member of that community seemed to develop a high level of trust by the larger society; a sense of 'doing the right things for the right reasons at the right time' in an evolving model of care for animals. If a case was brought into the hospital that required an unusual solution, we were usually allowed to do it and trusted to do our best.

Our mission statement was taken to heart by each staff member: "Extraordinary people providing extraordinary pet care twenty-four hours a day." We believed that if we did good, the absolute best we could for our clients and their pets, the rest would follow—including the financial aspects for continuing our work—and it did.

The two clinics grew and that very same year, a third hospital was purchased in Belfair, a community twenty miles from the original site. A young new partner, Dr. Gary Sleight, assumed the responsibilities of that endeavor. The year 1980 was a growing and thriving time—and extremely busy.

One night, sleeping on the floor of the office in my sleeping bag while being on call for emergency service, I thought to myself, this is ridiculous! I would have to get up early for cases the next day—I was not sure I could keep up this pace. So, as often happens in the middle of the night, an idea began to formulate: open a twenty-four hour practice at our large second hospital, with veterinarians and staff hired to serve the clients who needed evening and night hours, handle emergency night calls, and monitor hospitalized animals during the night. Again, we just did it. One office of the Central Valley Hospital was turned into a sleeping quarters and staff was hired to work the graveyard-shift hours. It was 1980 and we may have been one of the first twenty-four hour private veterinary practices in the nation. This concept became a successful endeavor and I got to sleep nights at home – important to my family now with three little boys in our home.

Idealism was allowed to soar, but idealism in a pragmatic world is difficult unless one has flexibility. As a private independent business, we had great flexibility to meet the needs of a diverse clientele and a great variety of animals. In the 1980s, a few veterinary specialists were found, most in the university setting, which for us was three hundred miles across the state. (Today, there are more than twenty-three specialty boards in our profession.) Veterinarians were, and still are, trained in the anatomy and physiology of all animals— except man. In those days, our hospital was simply expected to do it all: horses, dogs, cats, and wildlife. We often said, "If we can read it, we can do it." And we did.

The great diversity of animals that entered our hospital doors was a pivotal point of our growth and was an inspiration for our efforts; providing an underlying basis of joy to all the varied medical, business and cultural aspects of practice. There is no scientific study highlighting the percentage of unusual pets brought into a veterinary hospital, but needless to say, horses, dogs, cats and birds were the mainstay of our mixed clinical practice. Statistics cannot tell the complete story. Some of the most unusual 'pets' provide the most colorful portrayal of a veterinary practice. For instance, Goosey Gander was swaddled into our hospital.

The loud honker was a pet on a farm in the valley near our clinic. I assumed that the goose went after the neighbor's dog, knowing the protective personality of that feathered species. Unfortunately, the dog reacted with a quick snap to the beak and so, Goosey was brought into our hospital by a very distressed owner. Mrs. Neilson was sure to tell us that the gander was not just a roaming farm animal, but a true pet to the family. She rushed through the front door carrying her prized blanket wrapped goose under her arm and for once, the goose was quiet. Its lower bill was hanging in three pieces and the upper bill was missing the tip. The repair of a goose bill would not be found in a text book. Although veterinary education included a course in chicken pathology; goose anatomy and reconstruction surgery was not emphasized in class. With the severity of the injuries and the uncertainty of the repair, we were surprised that the owner wanted us to do whatever we could to return their goose to the farm.

After placing a tube down the trachea of the goose, gas anesthesia was administered (Fig. 20). Three veterinarians stood over the feathered patient discussing the best way to repair the bill. Our surgeon, Dr. O'Donnell, explained, "I can wire the lower jaw back together, as it is a boney projection, but I have no idea on how to repair the missing part of the upper beak." So, the first surgery our goose went through was a successful wiring of the bottom jaw pieces back together. Goosey woke up and appeared fine until we discovered he still couldn't eat due to the missing part of his top beak, which in bird anatomy is called the nail. The nail, or protruding tip of the beak, is important in grasping and rooting for food and, in this case, it was just plainly gone. There are times in a practice that a veterinarian will need to be creative in solving a medical or in this case, a beak-less problem.

Fortunately, one of our hospital's new veterinarians was a man of many talents: Dr. Ellithorpe was a talented artist in wood and bronze sculpture. His art work often depicted the animals and scenes of the natural wildlife environment. With specialized knowledge in animal anatomy, his sculptures created an extremely detailed and lifelike portrayal of wildlife animals.

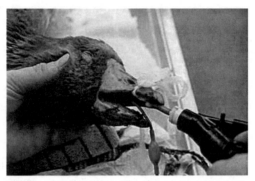

Figure 20:   Goosey Gander needs a new bill.

Ellithorpe toyed with the idea of sculpting an artificial end to the beak using an acrylic format. Acrylic material was kept at the clinic for hoof repair on horses, but it would create too much heat being applied and most likely would damage the existing goose beak tissues. Not to be deterred, a local dentist was approached who could provide us with an acrylic medium that is used in dental procedures. And thus, Goosey's tip of his beak was sculpted by an artist out of the dental acrylic material and then attached to the existing beak. Sound like a fairy tale? Maybe, but it worked. The wired jaw of his lower beak healed just fine and the new acrylic implant served Goosey well for the rest of his roaming goose life on the farm.

Appointments were just getting back to the 'normal' routine, when my receptionist came into the treatment room and announced there was a client on the phone who wanted to make an appointment for a wolf. Apparently the wolf, Gray Skies, had a problem with one of her eyes. She uncertainly asked, "What should I do?" She related that the owner had called several veterinarians in the area, but none wished to treat a wolf with a bad eye. One of the county's veterinarians had mentioned my expertise in animal eye cases. Maybe it was curiosity or a chance to work on a wolf's eye, but I accepted the appointment with a little trepidation. Later that afternoon, a long-legged wolf simply came walking into the hospital.

One doesn't quite get the true perspective of how big a wolf actually is, until one walks through your front door. She was a young wolf, but her feet were huge. The eyes and markings were distinct in nature's design. The client was built like a bear, reminding me of my father's logging days. There was a rope used for a leash, but she didn't lead very well. I never discovered how the client came to have a wolf as a pet.

Now, it must be said that other clients have brought what they called 'wolves' into the clinic, which in actuality were wolf-dog hybrids transported down from the North. A canid hybrid is a result from the mating of a dog and wolf. In 1998, it was estimated that there was 300,000 wolf-dogs in the United States. Many of these hybrids take on the behaviors of the dog, yet unpredictability would always be a concern. Today, according to the National Wolf-Dog Alliance, forty states forbid the ownership, breeding, and importation of a wolf-dog while others impose some form of regulation on ownership.

Gray Skies appeared entirely wolf-like, although she was rather timid in manner. She was holding her left eye closed. On approach, she didn't seem defensive or challenging. Before examining her, I wanted to remove any pain in the eye. Hopefully, without pain, she would hold her eye open for the exam. I only trusted the owner to restrain her, not wanting to expose my technician to any danger. Putting a drop of topical anesthetic into the light colored eye was without incident, only a slight normal dog-like jerk, which was reassuring.

While waiting for the anesthetic to numb the eye, I took a history of the injury from the client. The owner, Jeff Fosberg, indicated, "I was playing with Gray Skies in the grassy field behind our house, but when I brought her back inside, she was holding her eye closed." On first examination of the eye, I noticed an abrasion on the inside corner of her cornea. A sudden onset eye problem with an abrasion in that location is often caused by a grass seed behind the third eyelid. I was so hopeful for that particular diagnosis since treating it would not involve surgery or a stay in the hospital. With a muzzle in place around the strong jaws and the client firmly holding her head, I carefully lifted the third eyelid with forceps. To my good fortune, a large foxtail grass seed was clearly noticeable. Holding the third eyelid with one forceps and another forceps in the other hand, I teased the grass seed loose and removed it. The removal of the foreign body would be curative in itself. With a prescription for antibiotic ointment, Gray Skies was ready to go. Before they left, I asked if I could have a picture taken with her (Fig. 21). She was an exquisite animal, but I was certainly glad she was a young female wolf and the solution was straightforward.

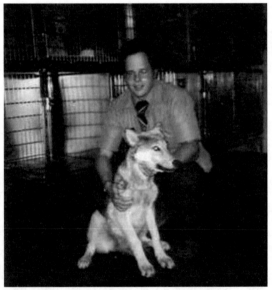

Figure 21: Gray Skies' eye problem

A diversity of animal species continued to enter our hospital doors. We were reluctant to treat primates in our hospital: they can sometimes be carriers of herpes B virus and tuberculosis, contagious to man. Again, an exception was made for a special case. Susa the Chimp was a young rising star in our community, with her owner planning to visit charitable children's events, nursing homes, and other nonprofit venues (Fig. 22). The State

Health Department said that since Susa could catch and carry childhood diseases she would need to be vaccinated pronto. Susa was brought in to the clinic for a complete physical examination, making sure she was healthy. The incredible strength and wiriness were noticeable in the long arms, but she had been well handled since she was young, making it easy to complete the exam. Finding her to be very healthy, vaccines obtained from the state were given to the little chimpanzee; only then did she seem to say, "Ouch!"

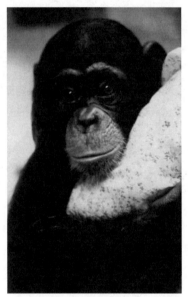

Figure 22: Susa the Chimpaneze

Emergencies arriving during appointment hours were given a name…show-stoppers. Show-stopper emergencies were so named because they could totally disrupt the morning or afternoon appointment schedule – and quite often did.

One show-stopper was unusual in that it involved an uncommon pet, a turtle, named Tilly. My receptionist interrupted a client's appointment time to inform me there was an injured turtle up front, one that had been run over by a lawn mower. A show-stopper, and with an apology to the client, I headed for the reception area to be greeted by outstretched hands bearing a turtle. "It's Tilly," he proclaimed, "I think she is dying." The injury was obvious, but not likely life threatening. There was a deep crack along the back of the shell where the lawn mower blade struck her (Fig. 23).

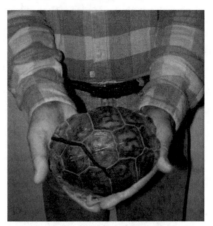

Figure 23:   Tilly's cracked shell

Mr. Johnsen gave a sigh of relief when I shared with him that she should be fine and the shell could be repaired. I asked him for permission to take Tilly to the back to be placed in a medical incubator, beginning treatment for shock and infection. Returning, I reassured him that Tilly would probably make a complete recovery. Mr. Johnson seemed much more relaxed and wanted me to know Tilly's history. "She is over 30 years old, handed down from my parents, and now our family pet. Tilly lives in an enclosed yard with a pond and spends her winters hibernating under our house. The spring grass in her enclosed area is long and I didn't see her till the mower blade struck her."

I went on to explain what would be necessary for Tilly's recovery. After shock and medical treatment, Tilly would need a 'cast' on her shell to stabilize the crack and promote healing. The 'cast' would consist of layers of fiberglass cloth glued together with a sticky resin. Mr. Johnson consented to the treatment.

Today, epoxy-impregnated fiberglass cloth and turtle-safe epoxies are recommended casting materials, but we did not have that option. Instead, we went to a local car body repair shop for fiberglass cloth and *Bondo* resin for our casting supplies. If we could think it, or read it, our surgeon, Dr. O'Donnell, could do it.

The following day, gas aesthesia was administered. The wound was cleaned, antibiotics continued, and the 'cast' applied. Tilly was visited in the hospital by neighbors, friends, and the whole family. She eventually went home to continue her long turtle life. Tilly was one of our many uncommon pets requiring a novel treatment solution – when putting pets first.

Animal humane work was part of every veterinary hospital's practice in those days. Good Samaritans often delivered injured or abandoned animals to a hospital for immediate care. That was the case of Little Hoot (Fig. 24). This big-eyed tiny owl was found along the side of the road, most likely hit by a car or had flown into a power line. Fractures were the most common reason that we treated birds of prey. Although frightened and appearing stunned, no external injuries or fractures were found on the owl's initial examination. The decision was made to give Hoot a warm and quiet place to recuperate overnight, hoping the shock would eventually wear off. After giving the supportive treatment, the little owl was definitely ready to go the next morning. Driving her to a secluded area, we released Little Hoot back into the forest. There is great satisfaction in treating wildlife and returning them to their natural habitat. The greatest reward of being a veterinarian is not monetary; it just feels good to help an animal…just to help an animal.

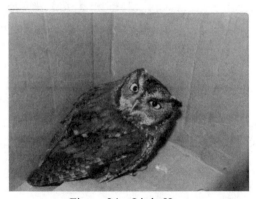

Figure 24: Little Hoot

Sometimes a Good Samaritan is misinformed as to how best to deal with an abandoned wildlife animal. In our Puget Sound setting, a young seal is often found 'abandoned' on the beach. Marine experts continually try to educate the local population that this situation can be a normal experience for a seal pup. In the autumn time, even though the seal pups can swim, the mother seal will put the seal pup on the beach and then go off to hunt. Later she will come back to get her pup. So, young seal pups may be left alone up to twenty-four hours. Unfortunately, people who find the pup on the beach simply assume something has happened to the mother and they need to rescue the abandoned and motherless pup. That is how our hospital staff became substitute parents of Web.

The two week old harbor seal was first found sitting on Lynch Cove near Hood Canal, a beautiful and natural marine environment. The people with good intentions who had found the abandoned pup were not sure what to do with it and called the State Game Department for advice. The state agency referred the seal to our hospital, since we were close to the area and one of our associates, Dr. Wayne Webster, had ties with the Marine Animal Resource Center in Seattle. The center provided medical care and found new homes for stranded or injured marine animals in the area. Web, named after Dr. Webster, became our first marine mammal patient.

Under the supervision of a certified marine veterinarian, we were allowed to provide rescue to this young seal. The marine center in Seattle was called on a daily basis for specific directions as to proper care. Our technician would go out to a local bridge to snag herring on a daily basis. Using a kitchen blender, the herring and baby food were pureed together for tube-feeding the little seal. It wasn't too long until little Web could eat full sized herring. Web was extremely intelligent, as well as an incredibly soft animal. After two months, he became very attached to the hospital's staff, following his favorites around in the clinic or playing out in the yard. The staff was fully enamored with the little pup. The seal's daily swim in the hospital's large bathtub was his favorite event, barking all the time (Fig. 25).

Web grew until just old enough for the Marine Animal Resource Center in Seattle to take him the following week end. At his late night feeding, he appeared to be fine, but one of our veterinarians had a funny feeling about Web in the night, and went down to check on the pup early the following morning. Web had died during the night. The entire hospital was devastated by the news. Since harbor seals are a protected species, Web was sent to the State Department of Fisheries for an autopsy. The pathologist of the department of fisheries later called us with the news that Web had died from sudden infant death syndrome, SIDS. It is an established diagnosis as a cause of death of young seals. Loosing any patient is difficult. Losing those you become personally attached to, regardless of species, is very difficult – as it was with Web. That is probably why most veterinarians don't treat their own pets with serious illnesses.

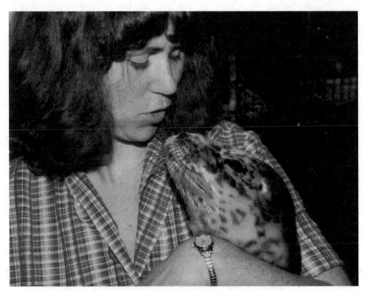

Figure 25: Web, the abandoned seal

I used to think there was nothing good about a raccoon, a bothersome pest from the forest or as something to decorate a Daniel Boone hat. In the Northwest, they are still often considered a neighborhood nuisance, raiding bird feeders and scavenging yards for food. So when a neighbor brought a litter of mother-less raccoons into the hospital, we questioned our role—for about a minute. What to do? One of the technicians, Michell, adopted the little raccoons, bottle feeding and tending to their needs. Dr. O'Donnell ended up taking all ten little ones home until they could fend for themselves, as they often caused chaos in the clinic. In the process we discovered their extreme intelligence and became enamored with their antics. After being released back in to the wild, one of the young came back to Dr. O'Donnell's porch after a year of living in the wild - almost knocking at the door. Her name was Seneca with a distinctive appearance, sporting a cowlick over one eye. She came and sat up on his lap, sharing a cookie with him. It was just to be a visit from a friend. Another one of the bottle-fed babes revisited his home on and off for over 14 years. Although the raccoon was visually impaired by cataracts, he would still come back for a cuddle. Raccoons are amazing animals.

The menagerie of wildlife that entered our hospital doors during this time of practice may be best summarized by an extraordinary species the Raptor Rehabilitation Center sent to our hospital for treatment. Our national bird, the bald eagle, had been shot in the elbow; it needed surgery. A pin was placed in the radius. The ulna, a large bone in bird anatomy, was plated. After a period of healing, the eagle was released on Fox Island. Watching it fly away was an unforgettable moment. Wildlife veterinary medicine is often challenging, but it is its own reward.

But…bills need to be paid. Horses, dogs, cats, and birds were the mainstay of our mixed clinical practice, providing the resources for our existence in the community. Although we never knew what was coming next through our front doors, most were cats and dogs.

On a particularly sunny Sunday afternoon, while covering emergency duty, I received a phone call from a dentist friend, Harold Sheldon. Sounding rushed, he said, "My dog Max is in trouble. He's retching terribly and I have no idea why." I told him to bring Max to the hospital and I'd be waiting for him.

The yellow Lab was obviously in distress, retching deeply and foaming at the mouth. While taking the history in the exam room, Harold seemed to have no idea what could have happened to Max. He had been hitting golf balls in the back pasture when his wife called him in to take a phone call. After about twenty minutes, he went back out to continue practicing his golf stroke. That is when he discovered Max in distress and called me.

My first thought was that Max may have a gastric torsion: a situation where the pet's stomach flips over while running. Usually the abdomen is extended in torsion, but Max showed no signs of extension. Being unable to make a diagnosis from the history, symptoms or physical exam, Harold agreed to an x-ray (Fig. 26).

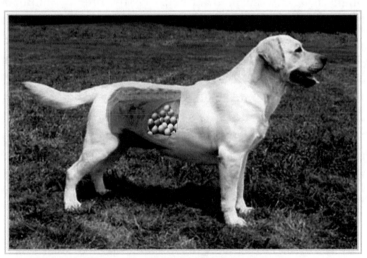

Figure 26: Max, the golf ball retriever

The radiographic finding was startling. I had never seen anything like this before. Max's stomach was chock full of golf balls. Rather than simply retrieving the balls, Max had swallowed each ball until his stomach could hold no more. Surgery retrieved thirteen golf balls, all in perfect condition for practicing a golf stroke…just not around Max.

There is a two gallon glass jar in my office containing many of the unusual objects taken out of the stomach of pets: fish hooks, rocks, baby bottle nipples, baby pacifiers, and the list goes on. Only keeping one golf ball for my collection, I gave a dozen golf balls back to the owner.

Dogs are not the only pets swallowing unusual non-food items. Cats have their share of strange situations. Kittens especially enjoy playing with a ball of string or yarn, which is fine unless they decide to eat it.

A small fluffy kitten named Bugs arrived on the exam table with a rather complicated string problem. When Mrs. Elton had arrived home from work, she noticed that the kitten had a piece of string hanging out of its mouth. She tried to tug it, assuming it would just pull free, but it didn't. Scaring her, she wisely brought it into the hospital for help. By the time I examined the kitten, it not only had string coming out the mouth but it was coming out the other end, as well. An x-ray showed that the kitten literally had string through her entire digestive system, from mouth to anus. One could not just ease the string loose; it was balled in the intestinal tract from end to end. Surgery was long, essentially making small slits in the intestines and removing small segments of the string. The de-stringed kitty recuperated well and was soon sent home after a few days in the hospital. Meanwhile, the client put her knitting and string in a high cabinet – no more 'strung-a-long' kitty would be allowed (Fig. 27).

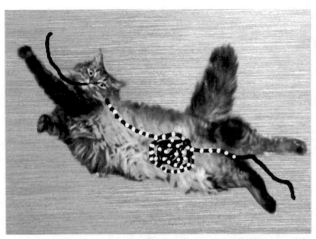

Figure 27: 'Strung-a-long' kitty

Sometimes, a pet can even open a drawer to find an unusual object for munching. Shasta, a white standard poodle, showed few symptoms on exam. On x-ray, there appeared to be a large balled mass within the stomach area (Fig. 28). Unable to decipher what the mass was other than a foreign body, exploratory surgery was needed. Upon opening the stomach, I was surprised to find that Shasta had eaten an entire set of intact panty hose. Later, when I returned the panty hose to the client, she sighed and explained, "I have a difficult time keeping Shasta out of my lingerie drawers." A rather unique case, but in this instance I refused the pantyhose for my foreign body collection jar.

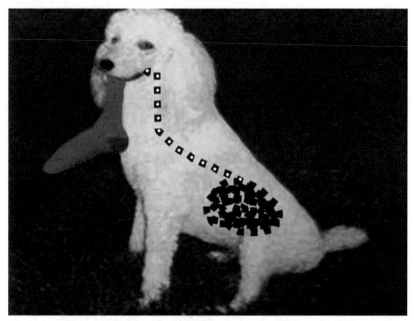

Figure 28:   Shasta's lingerie party

Meeting diverse cases and unusual situations made for extraordinary days in our veterinary practice. Being successful in meeting those challenges only continued to reinforce our new hospital's purpose.

The most common human-pet relationship remains the established family pet, whose role is primarily companionship. This in itself can benefit the family through the enjoyment of a social connection. There is another realm of the human-pet bond that includes companionship but goes beyond: the service animal. Service animals are truly extraordinary animals. We were fortunate to have many in our practice.

In the 1980s the most common service animals were the Guide dogs and the Police dogs. In times gone by Guide dogs were called 'seeing eye' dogs. Today, the role of the service animal has expanded into many different areas. Emotional support dogs help with depression and veterans with post-traumatic stress disorder (PTSD). Medical response dogs can detect low or high blood glucose with diabetics and bring a telephone or medicine as needed. A mobility service dog helps disabled individuals with gait and balance. They can open and close doors, and some have harnesses to pull wheel chairs. Hearing assistance dogs alert their owners to a variety of household sounds such as door knock or door bell, oven buzzer, telephone ringing, smoke alarm, and a baby crying. They will make physical contact with the owner and bring them to the sound. Seizure response dogs are a special type of service dog trained to help someone who has epilepsy or a seizure disorder. Other uses for service dogs are search and rescue, police work, bomb and drug detection and tracking. A special new field utilizing dogs is in cancer detection. It has been shown that, because of the unique smelling ability of the dog, they can detect with high accuracy patients with lung and bladder cancer. A special use of the human-pet bond is provided by the Pet Partners Program sponsored by the Delta Society. The program trains volunteers and screens volunteers and their pets for visiting animal programs in hospitals, nursing homes, rehabilitation centers, schools, and other facilities.

Cats and horses are not to be denied as service animals. Some cats can detect seizures hours before they happen, allowing the owner confidence to leave the house. Service cats help veterans with companionship and combat depression and post traumatic distress disorder. Therapeutic horse riding is extremely helpful for the disabled and those with special needs. It builds confidence, strength and coordination.

Service animals deserve the best. They were a high spot in our care for animals in the 1980s. Mr. Wilson was a distinguished older gentleman who was legally blind. His guide dog, a German shepherd named Scout, was referred to our hospital for an eye problem. His guide dog had developed degenerative pannus - a slow growing pigment, actually scar tissue, over the cornea. A blind man was faced with the possibility of having his guide dog going blind. To maintain the vision of the dog it was necessary to put drops in the eye three times a day. It wouldn't cure the problem, but would control it. The challenge was how to instruct him to effectively put drops in his dog's eyes. He lived alone, no other assistance other than his dog. Solution: for the few days necessary, I went to his house each morning and night to help him become independent in the procedure. He learned how much pressure to squeeze the bottle so the right amount of drops would be used. He practiced how to hold the dog's head still while administering the drops. He needed to be assured that the drops went into the eyes correctly. Scout was extremely cooperative, and his owner became very good at it. I only needed to monitor Scout's eyes periodically after that time. When a blind man's dog is going blind, everything that the profession can do will be done. These dogs are very valued because of their training, companionship and most importantly...for the work they do. The Guide Dogs of America is extremely supportive of veterinary care for their dogs.

Sometimes the owner can become a service person for their pet. Cleo, a three year old cocker spaniel, had been Mrs. Gilbert's emotional support through many difficult experiences. Cleo was definitely a service animal. Then the little dog developed primary glaucoma, first in one eye, eventually going blind in that eye. Then a few months later, the second eye was affected, in a gradually losing battle to retain vision. Cleo was blind and starting to develop severe pain; showing signs of hiding, just not being herself. Various means were attempted to control the pain, but the only certain way to address the severely degenerating eyes was to remove them. Before surgery I had prepared the client what to expect for a dog with no eyes. Upon the recheck visit, the client seemed delighted. She said, "Cleo is now like a puppy, bouncing around and playing. The pain must have been horrible." I asked her how Cleo was getting along being totally blind. I was totally surprised at her answer, "This dog has been my service animal for three years and now I am her seeing-eye person." Cleo continued to visit our hospital for routine visits for many years, and she was an amazing little dog.

Police dogs were, and still are, highly respected in our community. We worked with three different police departments in our area, caring for their law enforcement canine officers. In general, they came to the hospital for routine exams and preventative care. Being a twenty-four hour practice, flashing lights would herald an injured police dog. When we saw these service dogs for non-routine appointments it was usually in a very tense emergency situation--stab wounds or being shot in the line of duty. Quickly on the heels of the officers, news reporters and a film crew would arrive at our door. These dogs were public officers and given top priority in the news.

Riley was stabbed in the abdomen while on pursuit of a robbery suspect. The dog had been called in to find a fleeing suspect; trying to apprehend someone without putting an officer at risk. Besides, he was faster. The suspect was apprehended, but in the scuffle he had managed to stab Riley in the abdomen. The German Shepherd was hemorrhaging into his abdomen. He was bleeding out. During exploratory surgery, we found a lacerated spleen from the stab wound. The spleen needed to be removed. It was fortunate that organ was the only one affected by the knife and that he hadn't bled to death before surgery. Still, it was a big and time consuming job to remove Riley's spleen…there are so many vessels that have to be ligated. After close to three hours of surgery, Riley was finally allowed to recover in the surgical ward. All the news agencies awaited the outcome of the surgery at the hospital and pictures were taken as public record. Riley made a full recovery and actually went back into service after recuperation. The officers always stayed with the dog, no matter what was being done. These service dogs live with the family of their working officer and after retirement return to the family as a loved pet. Working with the police dogs was fascinating: they were the nicest dogs in the world, until they were put on command.

The 1980s were a busy, fulfilling decade. Our three veterinary facilities grew to nine veterinarians and forty support staff. The evening, emergency and extended weekend hours at the 24 hour hospital provided convenience and a level of care not previously available in the county. We could hardly keep up with the demand for our services. The profession's advancements in medical, dental, and surgical knowledge and techniques were rapidly accelerating. Combine all this with the deepening human-pet bond and increasing availability of specialty care made us change our thinking and by the early 1990s we could no longer comfortably say, "If we can read it in a journal or text book, we can do it." The era of veterinary specialty care and increased standards of practice had arrived. We were obligated to inform clients of specialty services if it was a complicated case, although most clients preferred us to provide the care rather than travel to Seattle or across the state to the veterinary college.

Realizing that more and more specialty services were on the horizon and the isolated nature of our county, we began adding equipment needed by specialists that we hadn't already purchased. Shortly thereafter we added the services of a veterinary dentist and an internist with cardiac patient experience to our umbrella practice.

With our day practice, extended hours, emergency services, and specialty care we were very likely one of the first private practices in the country to combine all these services in one delivery system. In spite of this growth, we never lost or forgot our private practice personality and values that allowed us the privilege of serving so many pets and clients.

Our service level, practice philosophy and flexibility allowed us to meet the needs of a diverse clientele and a great variety of animals, from pets to wildlife. We could still charge what was needed or exchange a service for a cord of wood if need be. I personally have never known a veterinarian who went into our profession for economic reasons. Veterinarians are idealists.... and these were our golden years. Our mission statement was lived: "Extraordinary people providing extraordinary pet care twenty-four hours a day." We believed that if we did good, the absolute best we could for our clients and their pets, the rest would follow—including the financial aspects for continuing our work—and it did.

It was a joyous time and place, we believed it would continue.

Chapter Five

It All Changed with a Phone Call

"Children and dogs are as necessary to the welfare of our country as Wall Street and the railroads."

-Harry S. Truman-

I write this book out of a necessity driven by a need to share practice case memories to illuminate the contrast to a currently fragmented veterinary pet care industry. In doing so, I hope to assist the modern day pet owner who is making veterinary care decisions for his/her pet. Professional idealism combined with meeting patient and societal obligations must be primary when recommending diagnostic testing, treatment options, and preparing cost estimates.

For purpose of illustrating the contrast between a James Herriot's *All Creatures Great and Small* style of veterinary medicine and the current small animal practice industry, let me repeat my historical background on how a small practice began, grew, and expanded by incorporating daily its values and personality.

After graduation at Washington State University's Veterinary College I accepted an internship with the Massachusetts S.P.C.A. Humane Hospital in Springfield, Massachusetts. During the fourteen month internship, we cared for thirty-one thousand patients, many of them sick or injured that were brought in by the Humane Hospital's rescue drivers. Maybe it was here, serving many of the inner city poor that further shaped my sense of professional idealism. It was here as an intern that I treated and cared for the many common forms of pet trauma and illness.

One thing I believed during my training is there must be more to pet eye care than either putting ointment in the eye or removing it. While looking for an opportunity to learn more about eye care, the medical director indicated that Ohio State University was the best place in the nation to learn about advanced animal eye care. Therefore I applied and was accepted into the animal ophthalmic training graduate program. Part of my time was at the human hospital in the department of ophthalmology, learning instrumentation by examining human patients with eye problems. That made it easier because humans, in difference to pets, would hold still. All in all, the learning couldn't have been better, but being a bit homesick and wishing to return to the Pacific Northwest, my wife and I loaded our worldly goods into our Volkswagen bug and with our standard poodle Travis, and our parakeet Petie, headed for home.

We settled into Tacoma and began an eye referral practice. The eye practice started slowly, but grew since I was, at that time, the only veterinarian in the Pacific Northwest with advanced eye training and necessary equipment. In a referral specialty practice, you seldom see the same client twice. After a year or so I decided to return to my home town, continue my eye care practice and add general small animal practice. I wanted to be a hometown veterinarian and see the same clients and pets on return visits.

Patty and I began our practice in 1973, on a financial shoestring. We were not initially listed in the phone book, so depended on family, friends, and my eye care practice to keep our doors open. The phone service started with two incoming phone lines. The first time we needed to put someone on hold and answer the other line was memorable. We called it our first double header. The office call fee at that time was five dollars. After just a few months and the business started to grow substantially, my receptionist called around and we raised our office call to six dollars. In those days, I didn't give itemized estimates. Instead, I would simple pick a reasonable dollar number and tell the client that the fee wouldn't be any more than that. For instance, a cat abscess would not exceed one hundred dollars or a given fracture would not exceed three hundred dollars. Sometimes I would need to adjust the invoice to stay within the dollar amount of those assurances given to the client. We often sent bills for our services if the client could put fifty percent down. I remember one year writing off twelve percent of the gross due to bad payment debts. It all worked, as practice growth was exploding, and we became so busy that sheer volume made up for our 'less than ideal' business practices. There were days when it was difficult to keep up with the practice challenges, both clinically and business wise, but it was all exhilarating. For early morning clients who couldn't leave work to make an appointment or when there were no more appointment slots available we provided a pet drop off service. As an illustration of the magnitude of our case load, I remember a day when all cages and kennels were full with a dozen or more drop-offs and I had to ask my receptionist for no more drop-offs until we could send some home.

I didn't begin with a business strategy of what was to happen; it just happened over the years to meet the needs to provide caring, comprehensive service for a constant growing demand. No matter what service we added that complimented our delivery of care, it became utilized and grew. I hope, by some of the stories I shared in earlier chapters, you can appreciate a special place and time. As a sideline, after about twenty years into the growth of the practice I looked at my personal yearly income tax return and remembered I had made more income in my early years practicing alone, but I wouldn't have traded ten times the income for what was to become for me the 'Shangri-La' of practice service: Serving nearly all of the pet care needs that came through the door with a flexible broad service level, a compassionate attitude and always conscious of a client's ability to pay for service.

By locating the practice in Kitsap County we were surrounded by the waters of Puget Sound. There were few specialty practices in Seattle in those early days. Referrals had to be made to the Veterinary College, 300 miles away in Pullman, Washington. It is little wonder that our un-fragmented, comprehensive and caring service grew and was unique in those early days compared to what was to become – a fragmented pet practice industry only further fragmented by the current consolidation efforts of national veterinary corporations. The present day pet care industry that I speak to means that many of the pet care services that used to be performed by your own local day care facility now involves traveling to various practice entities, i.e. specialists, emergency clinics, twenty-four hour hospital for monitoring and low cost or nonprofit humane services. Unfortunately, each one of these entities may have competing interests. Along with other changes within the profession in general, fragmentation of the veterinary pet care industry has resulted in ever-escalating fees for service, altered practice personalities and I hold, dimmed idealism, the primary reason we all became veterinarians.

To illustrate this fragmentation, I will use Kitsap County Washington, where I began my practice in 1973, in contrast with 2015. I believe there are similar national comparisons.

1973 Pet Practitioners and Facilities:
(County Pop. ~ 130,000)

Pet Practitioners:	**8**
Pets Exclusively	
Mixed - Pets and Livestock	
Practice Facilities:	**6**
Day - Pet Exclusively	
Mixed - Pets and Livestock	
*All did own emergencies / very few referrals	

2015 Pet Practitioners and Facilities: (County Pop. ~ 260,000)

Pet Practitioners: **55**
- Day
- Emergency
- Specialty
- Mobile
- Non-profit
- Military

Practice Facilities: 30
- Day Practices - Private Ownership
- Day Practices - National Corp. Ownership
- Emergency/Specialty Center-National Corp. Ownership
- Non-profit - Humane Society Ownership
- Military - U.S.Ownership
- Mobile - Private Ownership

With doubling of the population there are five times the number of small animal veterinary care facilities and seven times the number of small animal practicing veterinarians as when I began my practice in 1973. The traditional (do-it-all yourself) veterinary care facility with private ownership was the model in Kitsap county in 1973. By 2015, this model had fractured into an assortment of day, twenty-four hour, emergency, specialty, mobile, and nonprofit veterinary pet care facilities encompassing a mix of both private and national corporate ownership.

This fragmentation - accelerated by the entry of national corporations - gained even greater momentum by the mid 1990s, and was about to have a sudden and dramatic impact on our practice. It began with a phone call. The call began with a man stating his name and the company he represented. I had heard of the company before because of knowledge of their purchases of veterinary practices in the Seattle/Tacoma area. After introducing himself and his company, he asked me to join him for lunch. I thought since there were changes in the wind in the profession I thought I better listen to what he had to say.

Arriving at the restaurant, to my surprise two gentlemen dressed in suits introduced themselves and asked me to join them. I was a bit taken back by the formality of the situation. After introductions and some small talk, they indicated that their company was expanding into Kitsap County and wished to purchase our business and facilities. They seemed well informed concerning the facts and figures of what we had, as well as our general presence and growth in the county. They indicated they were in the process of purchasing other practices in the county and wanted to include ours. In a businesslike manner, one of the gentlemen said, "We wish to buy several veterinary hospitals in and around your county and develop a central facility." I indicated that I would discuss their proposal with my partners but didn't think we would be interested in their proposal at this time. With a few more words to clarify their intent and with a handshake, we left the restaurant.

I left the restaurant mentally numb as I realized I had been presented a difficult choice. Neither of my partners were initially interested in selling to the corporation. The thought of trading the known for the unknown was resisted. The corporate folks were persistent. Our biggest concerns were loss of our practice values, control of decision making, and who and how we would serve our clients and patients. Balancing against those concerns was the corporation's forward movement in buying practices, the assurances they provided to our concerns and their purchase price for business and equipment was tempting considering who would we sell to later if they carried out their strategy with the overwhelming investor resources they possessed. The corporation would retain all the employees along with providing them additional benefits. One of the partners could remain the medical director, if we wished, and we'd no longer need to address daily business concerns. After considerable partner hashing and rehashing, we sold to the corporate entity. Our youngest partner, for his share of the sale, kept one of the day practices. He wished to maintain practice autonomy.

My partner and I worked for the corporation for a few years. Without going into the details, our employment didn't work out. The need to conform to corporate policy often entailed 'biting my tongue.' Finally, with repeated insistence to adhere to strict protocols that effected how I practiced, I left. It was clear that the practice personality we sold would never be the same. It was time to semi-retire.

I began speaking on cruise ships during the winter and had part-time employment with my younger partner during the summer. All in all, it was a great career and I never along the way felt I sacrificed the reason why I became a veterinarian… that was to put the pet's needs first.

Chapter Six

Perspectives from the Kennel

"Lots of people talk to animals....not very many listen though... that's the problem."

-Benjamin Hoff, The Tao of Pooh -

Four years ago, I began writing this book. As a special interest speaker on cruise ships, I was often asked by passengers after sharing memories of patients I had helped, if I had a book. I thought maybe I should write down some of the memories on how and why I became a veterinarian, share a few stories to illustrate this special practice we had been, and what I thought pets and pet owners deserved from their veterinarian. For someone who had never written more than a term paper, I thought, "Author a book, me?" Anyway, with encouragement from family and friends - especially my wife - I began to write a memoir of how and why I became a veterinarian, the evolution of the human-pet bond, and reminisce on a special practice journey; sharing cases along the way. It would have to include the abrupt conclusion of the practice we had created. After writing the first four chapters, I thought maybe a publisher would be interested in my stories. I decided to submit the chapters to a few publishers. The first publishers sent me 'canned' email responses indicating no interest. Being a rather tenacious person, I sent to many more publishers. Again, they all rejected publishing my book but a few responses came with some scribbling with suggestions for the book. Consistently they indicated that I showed a love for pets and practice, but what they wanted to see beyond the memoir was a problem or problems that current pet owners face and proposed solutions. I wished initially to write the book as a memoir and illustrate the ever evolving human-pet bond I witnessed from my childhood days and how it would influence the future pet care industry. Now, with a stack of rejection notices and no 'client problem' that I could identify, I set my book aside hoping to come back some day to finish for my family.

In full retirement I had the time and nagging, compelling desire to finish my book. My practice stories were written, hopefully interesting and at times humorous, as a memoir in a time and setting of an ever strengthening human-pet bond. Out of that strengthening of the bond, in the 'do-it-all yourself' era of pet practices the veterinary pet care industry added a diverse group of highly competent niche practices, i.e. emergency and specialty. They developed from a growing desire by pet owners to protect that special bond. Entering recently into the fragmented delivery system, came investors with practice consolidating strategies along with strict business and accounting practices.

Recognizing the changes within the veterinary pet care industry, my personal struggle with diminished idealism within our profession, concerns from many pet owners, and finally, a conversation at a recent family reunion, compelled me to finish the book.

These concerns, both from clients and personally, cannot be separated from some current troubling veterinary practice industry realities. To not mention these realities would do disservice to understanding the origin of pet owners' concerns. My intent for briefly touching upon them is to more clearly shed light on how these concerns evolved. Without going into details, the following titles of a few articles in recent veterinary periodicals will provide an overview of current realities for the small animal practitioner. Some of the current titles: *Too Many Veterinarians or a Bubble Market; ? Falling Demand Trap New Vets.; Pros and Cons of Private Versus Corporate Practice; FTC Pushes for More Competition in Pet Medication Market; General Practitioners Vs Specialists: Competition and Collaboration; The Feminization of Veterinary Medicine; Vets- yet another Profession Suffering from Delusional Grads; High Suicide Rate Among Veterinarian; There is Not Enough Work for Veterinarians; Veterinary Non-profits: Unfair Competition or Worth Charities?* These topics highlight some of the stresses facing veterinary pet practice practitioners in a time when the cost of doing business continues to escalate, while for many, the number of office visits is waning.

These practice realities, in my opinion, have played a significant role as a catalyst for the concerns many pet owners experience in the current veterinary pet care delivery modality. I would not begin to suggest solutions to the multiple realities veterinary pet practitioners struggle with on an ongoing basis – the market place will sort them out. I do feel that in the future there will be more consolidation of large private veterinary practices by national corporations. Therefore, there will be fewer large privately owned veterinary practices. Also, there will be fewer small day practices, as their owners in the future will find a limited number of buyers for their practice and facility. There will be more and larger nonprofit corporate practices as well as low-cost alternatives for sources of affordable veterinary pet care. These changes and other shifts in practice size and ownership, with the ongoing industry consolidations, will alter specialty and emergency practices as well. I find it a bit ironic that the solo small animal mobile practice is emerging. Their ability to provide quality medical care, flexibility with medical decisions, competitive fees, and a high level of client bonding is refreshing.

Turning to client concerns, a conversation with my wife's cousin at a recent family reunion brought these many concerns into focus. Mary's regular veterinarian, a solo practitioner, was treating her dog for epilepsy. He felt a larger practice would be better equipped to monitor and address any possible future seizures. Mary made an appointment at the other practice.

A blood test was performed and medication prescribed. Once home she thought the prescribed medication seemed quite expensive and compared its price to the same medication, same amount from her previous veterinarian. To her surprise it was twice as expensive, yet she felt comfortable with her pet's care. At about the same time it became necessary for this particular pet's annual wellness examination. She thought, since the pet was being monitored for epilepsy at the new clinic, she would return to the same clinic for the wellness examination. During the exam many additional tests that she was unfamiliar with were recommended. She agreed because the veterinarian was certain that these preventative considerations needed to be addressed now. Samples for testing were taken and she was asked to call later for test results. Upon reaching the front desk she was presented a bill for the wellness examination and extensive testing for $470. The pet's previous wellness exam and tests at her original veterinarian office had been $160. After she went home and examined the bill, she felt she had been over marketed to and oversold, in other words, a sense of being overcharged. From that point on she made a decision she would have any future care for her pets done with her previous veterinarian.

This experience highlights the most common concerns, not having to do with competency, but linked to either cost, inflexibility or an issue of trust. I share Mary's concerns; not to disparage anyone or any service, but after years of listening to clients concerns, Mary's conversation and what I perceive as withering professional idealism, I was further motivated to finish my book.

But what about you and the veterinary care for your beloved pet? In listening to clients concerns over the years, they seem to fall into three categories: those being affordability (many people are unhappy with veterinary pet care because of cost), inflexibility (strict protocols dictating treatment and fees) and diminished trust. After pondering solutions to these various areas of clients concerns, these are my recommendations.

First, educate yourself and be informed concerning the preventative (vaccinations and parasites) and wellness needs of your particular pet. These needs vary by age, where you live, and how your pet spends its time. A hunting dog's preventative care is much different than a dog kept in an apartment. An indoor/outdoor cat has infectious disease risks much higher than one that lives exclusively indoors. An indoor cat's life expectancy is at least fifteen years. In comparison, cats that spend part of their time outdoors have an average life expectancy of seven years.

Second, with an illness concern, after a thorough history and physical examination are performed, a diagnosis at that time may be given. If the diagnosis is unable to be stated, ask for a list of tentative diagnoses and the best way to differentiate them to a definitive diagnosis. For example, if a pet is presented with frequent vomiting and the abdomen is palpated detecting a foreign body, one can be fairly certain it is the cause of the vomiting. That diagnosis often can be confirmed with an x-ray. If no diagnosis can be made from the history and examination, then a list of tentative diagnoses can be presented. Rather than performing a multitude of tests, what is the most likely diagnosis and what test would confirm it? With that diagnosis or tentative diagnosis, go online and look it up. You'll be pleasantly surprised at the amount of information available for a specific condition. With a given diagnosis or tentative diagnosis, always ask to be educated about all the options available. One of those options is always a second opinion. A second opinion, if time allows, can be reassuring during your decision process.

Third, your pet's medical needs often do not lend themselves to your veterinarian's day practice office hours. Research your emergency care options, in case an emergency concern should occur after hours. This applies equally to knowing the specialty care options in your area. Always ask to know all options with emergency or specialty care.

Fourth, when in need of expensive or long term pharmaceutical medications that are prescribed, it is entirely feasible to go to an online pet pharmacy and compare prices. If the price highly favors the online pet pharmacy, ask your veterinarian for a prescription and have it filled online or often now at human pharmacies. If asked, most veterinarians will provide a written prescription. Human medical offices don't fill a prescription for their patients, they write them and one can shop around. Non-prescription medications and products are readily available at box-store retailers at competitive prices.

Fifth, your veterinarian has an unlimited number of tests, procedures, products, and services in his/her professional toolbox. As a famous President once said in a different context, "Trust, but verify." Nothing could be more pertinent advice for addressing the concerns clients have expressed to me over the years. Being informed and proactive, your pet's health and your family budget will both benefit.

These recommendations for your consideration are intended to address concerns and serve as a road map through the realities that are changing the veterinary pet care industry of today. If nothing else, my perspective from the kennel opens up a conversation, but the health and well-being of your pet is the focus of my journey.

Putting your pet first is nothing new. It is a veterinarian's patient and societal obligation encapsulated within the veterinary oath. After all, compassion is the foundation of the veterinary profession.

Biographical Sketch

Dr. John Sleasman, DVM

John Sleasman, DVM is an experienced practitioner on the unique subject of veterinary medicine. His forty years of practice provides a revealing, humorous, and educational viewpoint of the universal love of the family pet. His experiences highlight the remarkable bond between humans and pets.

John was born and raised on the Kitsap Peninsula of Washington state. After earning a degree at Washington State University in Veterinary Medicine, being chosen to further his education with an internship with the Society of Prevention of Cruelty of Animals at Rowley Memorial Hospital in Springfield, Massachusetts, and graduate work in animal eye problems at Ohio State University, he returned to his home state to open a veterinarian practice. The small clinic grew into three hospitals on the Kitsap Peninsula, providing a standard of care unique to the world of family pets. Continuing education provided certification as a Veterinary Board of Veterinary Practitioners in feline and canine species. In retirement, being a cruise ship special interest speaker provides John the opportunity to continue his lifelong commitment to helping pet owners and their beloved pets.